NCT Book of

Child Health

Dr Morag Martindale

Thorsons

An Imprint of HarperCollins*Publishers*
in collaboration with National Childbirth Trust Publishing

Thorsons/National Childbirth Trust Publishing
Thorsons is an Imprint of HarperCollins*Publishers*
77–85 Fulham Palace Road
Hammersmith, London W6 8JB

Published by Thorsons and
National Childbirth Trust Publishing 2000

1 3 5 7 9 10 8 6 4 2

© 2000 NCT Publishing

Dr Morag Martindale asserts the moral right to
be identified as the author of this work

Illustrations: Jo Dennis

A catalogue record for this book
is available from the British Library

ISBN 0 7225 4014 0

Printed and bound in Great Britain by
Caledonian International Book Manufacturing Ltd, Glasgow

Contents

The National Childbirth Trust (NCT) offers information and support in pregnancy, childbirth and early parenthood, and aims to enable every parent to make informed choices. The NCT is working towards ensuring that its services, activities and membership are fully accessible to everyone.

Donations to support our work are welcome.

About the author

Morag Martindale is a GP and family planning doctor working on Tayside. She has three children and joined the National Childbirth Trust during her second pregnancy. She is currently involved at a regional level as area representative for Tayside and Fife. She is also a member of the Tayside Joint Breastfeeding Initiative.

Introduction

Caring for our children covers every aspect of their daily lives, especially those days when they don't feel very well. At these times they'll need extra amounts of loving attention, cuddles and comfort, as well as the appropriate medical treatment.

Healthy, lively children still routinely catch minor illnesses and sometimes more serious diseases too. There will always be a certain number of bugs, colds and infectious ailments doing the rounds but fortunately the vast majority do not pose a problem. Knowing when to treat them yourself and when to call in the doctor is important.

This book is intended as a quick reference guide, to help you find the best remedy for your child's complaint quickly.

Dr Morag Martindale
January 2000

1

Recognising illness

When a child becomes ill, parents are naturally worried. Even a mild temperature can cause a child to be listless and sleepy and it becomes quite obvious, even to a new parent, that their child is not well. In the days of extended families living in one house or at least very close to one another there was often another parent around who had been through it all before and could give advice and reassurance. These days this is less common; often you are on your own, or with a partner who is as inexperienced as you are, so dealing with a sick child can be frightening.

Don't forget that all children get ill. No matter how well you care for your child, all babies and young children will inevitably fall prey to ailments. In fact, it can sometimes seem as though the early years are a continuous round of coughs, colds and minor infections. It helps to stay calm: a mother's mood has a strong affect on her baby and although it can be difficult to keep from being worried and irritable when nursing a sick child (as well as weary from lack of sleep), remember that children generally bounce back very quickly.

Here are some guidelines to help you cope.

Fevers

If anyone your child has been in contact with has been ill with a cold or virus, then the child may well have the same thing. Colds, sore throats, ear infections and tummy bugs all usually have short incubation periods of just a few days (an incubation period is the time between catching the illness and the signs or symptoms appearing). The childhood fevers such as chickenpox often have longer incubation periods: these are all listed in the separate section later in the book. Urine and kidney infections, which are not usually passed from one person to another, will cause a raised temperature.

A symptom is what you complain of to your doctor and a sign is what the doctor looks for on examination. One of the first signs of illness in a child is a raised temperature. Your child's skin may feel warmer than usual to touch and the child's face might be flushed, so start by taking your child's temperature.

How to take your child's temperature

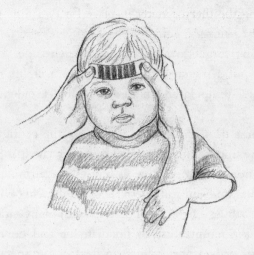

A 'Fever Strip' placed against the child's forehead will give a quick estimate of his or her temperature.

Other reliable methods of checking your child's temperature are with a mercury thermometer or an ear thermometer. Ear thermometers are relatively expensive, so although they do give a very quick and accurate reading it is worthwhile learning to read a mercury thermometer. Mercury thermometers are available from any pharmacist.

First of all shake the mercury down towards the bulb. Hold the thermometer at the end opposite the bulb and shake it down. To read the thermometer you will need to rotate it slightly and look for the level of the mercury.

Try this before you need to, so that you know what you are doing. If you still have problems reading the thermometer ask your practice nurse or health visitor to show you. You will need to keep shaking it down until the mercury is about 35°C or less. Now place the bulb end under the armpit and cuddle your child towards you, keeping the thermometer in place for two minutes. Then read it again.

Don't forget to shake it down each time you use it. Don't put a mercury thermometer in a child's mouth to read her temperature in case the child accidentally bites it.

These days doctors and nurses use the centigrade scale and the upper limit of normal is usually taken as 37°C.

A normal temperature is always reassuring but if the child has one and still doesn't seem right, check it again in a little while. The normal pattern with many viral illnesses is for the temperature to fluctuate up and down for the first day or two of the illness, prior to more specific symptoms developing. The aim of treatment of a fever is to keep the temperature as normal as possible during this period. This is done with paracetamol – either as a syrup or dissolving tablets or, in cases of severe vomiting, paracetamol suppositories inserted into the back passage.

Paracetamol treatment should be accompanied by tepid sponging. To do this, remove all of the child's clothing except the nappy. Take a bowl of lukewarm water and a flannel or sponge and sponge the child all over. The water should evaporate on the skin, so don't dry with a towel. If the temperature is very high you can speed up the evaporation by fanning with an electric fan or even a newspaper. Be warned that your child will not like it! However, it is very important that you do this continuously until you succeed in lowering the temperature. In an acute feverish illness you will find that the temperature will start

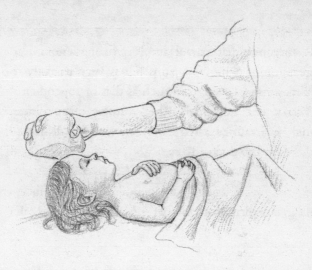

to go up again within a few hours and you will need to start the process all over again.

When treating a fever with paracetamol, always follow the instructions on the bottle and give paracetamol in the dose recommended for the age of the child.

Never run out of paracetamol. Children often become ill at night so make sure your medicine cabinet is stocked up.

Repeat the dose. Paracetamol will last at best for 6 hours but usually for 3–4 hours. Don't exceed the recommended dose for a 24-hour period as shown on the bottle.

Never wait for a doctor to come before giving paracetamol. Children may seem normal an hour after a dose of paracetamol, even when they were quite unwell before. This is often why they seem better as soon as the doctor arrives! However, doctors want to assess the illness, not the fever, and it is often easier for a doctor to assess a child who has had paracetamol.

Remember that paracetamol is strong enough to treat minor aches and pains but is very unlikely to mask a more severe pain such as that of appendicitis. Also it will not mask other features of an illness, such as a rash or a red eardrum, which will still be there for the doctor to see.

Don't give aspirin to the under 12s. Paracetamol is safer.

Aspirin, when given during a fever in young children, has been linked to a serious illness called Reye's syndrome. Although it is very rare, it is not worth taking the risk when paracetamol is so much safer and just as effective.

Give plenty of fluids. If you have ever had a fever yourself you will know that it affects your appetite. We can all, even young children, cope for a few days without our normal food intake. We cannot cope without water, however, and a fever means that we lose even more by sweating, so drinks in any form will do. Keep rehydration powders handy (e.g. Dioralyte). These are flavoured, usually come in sachets and are made up with cooled, boiled water. They are designed to replace the salts that are lost. However, many children do not like them because of their slightly salty taste. Try letting them drink through a straw. They won't taste so much this way!

They are important because they help the gut to absorb water. It's really important to keep fluid intake up.

Be prepared to nurse your child during the night if need be. His temperature will fluctuate up and down.

Don't drink alcohol when your child is ill. Apart from the fact that you need your wits about you, you may need to drive your child to an out-of-hours centre or hospital accident and emergency (A&E) department.

Avoid wrapping your sick child up in blankets. Keep the room reasonably cool and make sure the child is in light clothing.

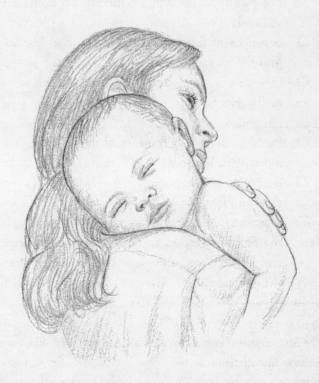

Other signs of illness

As well as a fever there are other signs of illness to check for and inform your doctor. These are serious and need immediate attention:

- ❏ child is off feeds (less than half of normal in last 24 hours)
- ❏ persistent vomiting
- ❏ fast breathing rate especially if the breathing is noisy and the breathing difficulty has come on suddenly
- ❏ fewer than four wet nappies in the last 24 hours
- ❏ the child is sleepy at a time of day when normally alert
- ❏ irritability
- ❏ blood in the bowel motions or in the urine
- ❏ a persistent unusual cry
- ❏ listlessness or floppiness
- ❏ the child is very pale
- ❏ delirium – if the temperature is very high the child may seem to be in a sort of a trance and even see things which aren't there (hallucinations).

Contact your doctor without delay. See pages 13 to 16 for more information.

Rashes

A rash is a crop of spots.

Skin rashes can be caused by infections or allergies or by diseases which affect the skin such as eczema.

An infection-related rash will usually be accompanied by a fever and signs that the child is ill such as catarrh or being off-colour.

An allergy-related rash may produce a mild fever but this is rare. The child usually appears very well and this rash is often intensely itchy. It may take the form of red spots which seem to run into each other, or urticaria which may look like a nettle rash or have raised blotches with paler centres.

Skin disease rashes, unless there is a complicating infection, will not usually be accompanied by a fever. Eczema is also itchy but the skin is often obviously dry. See the section on childhood fevers on page 79 for the characteristics of the main infectious childhood illnesses and also the sections on urticaria (page 165) and eczemas (page 108).

Doctors make a diagnosis based on the features of a rash. These are:

❏ *The length of time the rash has been present*
Spots that have been present for days with no sign of a fever when a child is clearly bouncing with health will probably be due to a non-infectious skin condition. For example, if the spots are in the areas which sweat, such as the front of the chest or the armpit, they could be a simple heat rash. Spots in the crook of the elbow or behind the knees may be eczema. The exceptions are infestations such as scabies, which are infectious.

Spots which have just appeared, especially when accompanied by a high temperature, are most likely to be one of the childhood fevers. In the early hours of these illnesses the spots may look the same, so if you decide to take your child to the surgery early on don't be surprised if your doctor is not absolutely certain of the diagnosis. You may be asked to go back after 24 hours to confirm it.

❏ *The type of spots*
Doctors group spots according to what they look like. *Macules* are flat red spots. *Papules* are red spots raised a little off the skin. (Measles spots, for example, are described as maculopapular; i.e. some are flat and some are raised, but they are all red!) *Vesicles* are blisters – the typical

chickenpox rash is vesicular. (However, just to confuse you, the blister may take a little time to develop, so to start with the spots may be maculopapular.) The most worrying kind are the purpuric spots. These are the spots of meningitis. The big difference here is that they do not blanch. If you press the side of a clear drinking glass firmly onto the spots or bruises they will not fade. See Meningitis on page 139. You must get a doctor's opinion immediately if you are confronted with this type of spot.

❏ *The area of the body covered by spots*
Chickenpox spots tend to affect the trunk and head although a few may appear on the limbs. In measles or rubella the limbs are also affected. In hand, foot and mouth disease the spots affect the hands, feet and mouth! They also extend up the backs of the legs and sometimes onto the buttocks.

❏ *Other symptoms which may accompany the spots*
The spots of an infectious illness commonly appear a few days after the child has been noted to be generally unwell. A parent may have noticed that the child seems clingy, is off food and possibly feverish. The advent of spots often confirms the diagnosis.

❏   *The numbers of spots*

Chickenpox spots occur in crops, with more appearing every two days or so until there are dozens. The rashes associated with the other childhood fevers also produce large numbers of spots. In contrast, molluscum contagiosum, a harmless viral infection which can be confused with chickenpox, see page 144, may produce from only one or two spots to a crop of 20 or more.

Many of the above symptoms will result simply from a fever and so you should treat the child's fever immediately. Fever is often the first sign that an illness has begun but it can be 24–48 hours before the signs appear which enable a doctor to make a diagnosis. This is why doctors often do not give antibiotics at the start of an illness, even when a child seems quite ill. Once your doctor knows what is causing the fever, and if it is something which responds to antibiotics, then it is safe to treat.

2

When to call the doctor

Don't forget that you can call your doctor or nurse if you are really worried about your child. If you do, be prepared to give as much information as possible. Your doctor will have a list of calls to make to sick patients and it is vital that he or she has enough information to make a decision on who needs to be seen first. Always try to make sure that the person phoning has some information about how serious the case is.

Unless there is no alternative, don't ask a child to make the call. Children find it difficult to give a proper assessment of the degree of urgency of a call and emergency staff are likely to err on the side of caution and treat a child's call as urgent even if it is not.

The ambulance service is there for the acute emergencies which need immediate transport to hospital and as a back up when your doctor is attending an emergency elsewhere. When you dial 999 you will first be asked which service you require. When you are connected to the service the first thing that happens is that you will hear your telephone number being repeated. You can then give details to the ambulance control officer, who will tell you when an ambulance will be available and what to do in the meantime. If the officer feels that a doctor will be needed he or she will contact your own doctor or the nearest surgery. All calls to the ambulance service and calls to many emergency doctor services are recorded.

Nowadays parents are often expected to take their child to a health centre or a hospital accident and emergency (A&E) unit to see a doctor out of hours. Many people worry that taking an ill child outside at night might make the child's condition worse. This is not the case and it is likely to be better for the child to be examined in a health centre with all the equipment the doctor is likely to need, not least good examination lighting, than at home.

Dial 999 for:

❏ anyone who is unconscious
❏ anyone who has severe bleeding
❏ choking not responding to first aid
❏ accidents where there are head or neck injuries
❏ fractures (unless involving wrist, hand or foot when the child is otherwise well)
❏ acute poisoning.

Contact your doctor immediately for advice if there is a child with:

- ❏ severe breathlessness
- ❏ allergic reactions with urticaria and facial swelling
- ❏ neck stiffness/sensitivity to light/purpuric rashes
- ❏ repeated vomiting and diarrhoea
- ❏ a temperature greater than 39°C not responding to paracetamol and tepid sponging
- ❏ unexpected drowsiness and listlessness
- ❏ abdominal pain not responding to paracetamol
- ❏ convulsions with no previous history, or a convulsion lasting longer than a minute.

The doctor or nurse on duty will tell you what to do.

Go to hospital casualty department for:

- ❏ suspected wrist/hand or foot fractures
- ❏ cuts that you think need stitching
- ❏ eye injuries
- ❏ accidental poisoning (phone first for advice).

Whether you should call 999 or take your child straight to Accident and Emergency may depend on the area in which you live. For example, in some you would dial 999 and in others you would go straight to hospital casualty in a case of poisoning. When you dial 999 the ambulance crew is obliged to take you to the nearest Accident and Emergency (A&E) unit. They cannot take you to your doctor's surgery or anywhere else. Before you need to, make sure that you know where your nearest A&E is and check that they have the facilities there to treat children.

Note that if you are a UK resident you are entitled to free medical care in any doctor's surgery or NHS hospital if you are on holiday in the UK. Non-UK residents are entitled to emergency care.

3

Giving medicine to your child

Once you or your doctor have decided that your child needs to have medicine it is important that your child takes it. Many children don't like medicine in spite of the fact that pharmaceutical companies try to make children's medicines taste as nice as possible.

If you find that your child does not like paracetamol syrup, try every brand. If all else fails, buy dissolving tablets and dissolve them in a small amount of a drink which you know your child likes. The key words here are 'a small amount'. If you dissolve the tablets in the child's drink make sure the child drinks it all; otherwise you will not know how much has been taken.

Many medicines, including paracetamol, are made in a sugar-free formulation to help to protect the teeth from decay. Always ask your pharmacist if one is available. For the same reason it is a good idea to brush your child's teeth after each dose.

Most over-the-counter medicines are supplied in a pack with full instructions and a list of possible side effects. It is necessary to list every side effect which has ever been linked to the drug, which can be alarming. However, be reassured that our drug licensing laws are among the strictest in the world and are particularly stringent for medicines manufactured for children. Read the list and if you have any concerns, ask your pharmacist.

It is extremely important that medicines, whether prescribed or over the counter, are taken according to the instructions. If medicines are required to be taken several times a day many people find it difficult to remember when each dose was taken and even if it was taken at all! If you are nursing a sick child you may be too preoccupied to remember exactly when you last gave a drug, so write it down.

Always finish a course of antibiotics unless your child develops side effects to it. A rash starting just after the course has been started may indicate that the child is allergic to that particular antibiotic and if so it will need to be stopped immediately. Always keep a note of the names of such drugs for future reference. The child may seem better within a day or two of starting treatment. However, the length of courses of antibiotics has been worked out to ensure that bacteria are killed off and an illness may recur if you stop the treatment too early.

You may have some over-the-counter medicine such as paracetamol left over after the child is better. Keep it in the fridge until the next time it is needed, but always check the date. Every drug should have an expiry date marked clearly on the pack or bottle. Never use out-of-date drugs.

Special syringes are available to make it easier to measure and administer medicine to babies and children.

With one hand cuddle your child towards your chest and with the other place the end of the syringe in the child's mouth. Wait until your child opens her mouth and tip the medicine on to her tongue. You may need to tip her chin up slightly with the same hand to make sure that she doesn't spit it out.

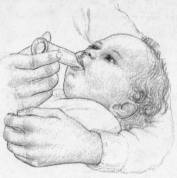

Eye drops

If your child has conjunctivitis you will need to administer eye drops or ointment. Children do not like having drops put in their eyes so you will need to have patience! It is easier if there is another adult to help you. One adult can cuddle the child, keeping her arms by her side, while the other gently turns the lower eyelid down and squeezes either the drops or ointment on the inside of the lower eyelid. This is easier than it sounds because it only takes a tiny amount of the drops to dissolve in the tears to enable the drop to spread all over the eyeball. It may seem that most of the dose has come out again, especially when the child blinks, but don't worry about this because enough will stay in. Giving eye drops is trickier if you are on your own – I have in the past resorted to giving drops to a child who is asleep!

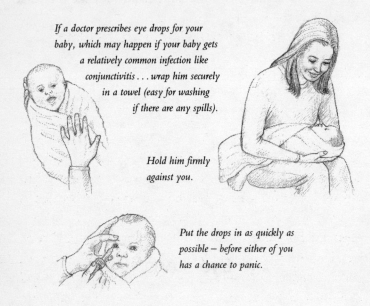

If a doctor prescribes eye drops for your baby, which may happen if your baby gets a relatively common infection like conjunctivitis . . . wrap him securely in a towel (easy for washing if there are any spills).

Hold him firmly against you.

Put the drops in as quickly as possible – before either of you has a chance to panic.

Ear drops

Ear drops are fairly straightforward and do not usually cause discomfort, so children are not normally upset by them. If you give your child a firm cuddle, keeping the arms in with one arm, you will find it easy to give the drops with the other hand.

4

Nursing your child at home

When your child is ill he will not feel up to playing or his other usual activities. He will appreciate being allowed to rest on a sofa or chair so that he is near you. This way, it will also be easier for you to keep an eye on him. Make a 'nest' for him on the sofa with his own pillows and toys. Let him sleep if he needs to and give him plenty of cuddles and extra attention. Keep a drink close at hand and don't worry about food. He will regain his appetite when the illness is over. Don't wrap a feverish child up in lots of blankets and duvets. He needs to be kept cool.

If your child has to be admitted as an emergency to hospital, you will not have much time to prepare him for it. Unless there is no alternative you should try to go with him and stay as long as you can. Most children's units have parents' rooms and you may be able to sleep beside him if he has his own room. He will be very frightened and will be reassured if you are there.

If he is going into hospital for a planned operation you will have time to prepare him for it. Some children's units will allow children to visit the ward prior to admission. He will be able to see that there are lots of toys and that the nurses are kind and helpful. This helps to allay anxiety about admission. Ask the nurse at the out-patient clinic if this is possible and make sure that you are clear yourself about what will happen. Talk to your child about it beforehand. You will normally be allowed to stay with your child right up to the time of the operation, perhaps even going in to the anaesthetic room if you wish. Special teddies or comfort blankets will usually be allowed into the anaesthetic room and recovery room.

When your child is admitted to the ward a nurse will take details of the medical history. Just as important are special instructions on any dietary likes/dislikes, religious or cultural issues relating to the stay in hospital and other things such as your child's way of indicating that he needs to go to the toilet.

Children are usually very sleepy after an anaesthetic, sometimes for several hours. You will probably want to be there when he wakes up to reassure him. He may be in pain and again the ward staff should tell you in advance how this will be handled. Many wards work a 'named nurse' system. One nurse is assigned to be the first contact person for you and your child and their name should be noted by the bed.

Nowadays adults and children alike are discharged from hospital much earlier than they used to be. You should be given instructions on what to expect at home and under what circumstances you should contact your doctor.

Complications are rare but one of the commonest is wound infection. If the wound site becomes red, hot or swollen, or if your child develops a temperature, you should contact your doctor right away. In some areas where early discharge is usual, specially trained nurses from the hospital visit at home in the early days to check that all is well.

As soon as a child is well again he will want to get up and play. If there are any instructions (e.g. on weight bearing after an orthopaedic operation) you should be told. Otherwise allow him to get up if he wants to. Children do not fake illness and will bounce back as soon as they are ready.

5

Coping with accidents

This chapter covers simple first aid procedures. However, it is no substitute for real training and it's always a good idea to attend an accredited first aid course. Never hesitate to telephone 999 if you think it is necessary.

Every house should have a first aid kit. It should be kept out of the way of small children but stored somewhere convenient and easily accessible. Overleaf you will find a list of items which your first aid kit should contain. All should be available from your pharmacist.

The list is divided into those items which the author believes should be in every first aid kit and those which are also useful but not absolutely essential. Don't forget to check your first aid kit now and again and replace missing or out of date items.

Essential items:

- a pad to stop bleeding, such as a gauze swab
- a bandage to hold the pad on if you are on your own. Bandages can also be used for other less urgent cases such as sprains
- a pair of scissors – blunt on one of the outer surfaces – to cut clothing, also useful to cut bandages and pads
- protective gloves. You may have to use your first aid kit for a stranger who is bleeding. The gloves will protect you from infection
- for the same reason, a mouth mask for mouth-to-mouth resuscitation. This can be a quite simple device and does not need to be expensive. Such masks are available for first aid kits and as keyrings
- a thermometer
- paracetamol in formulations to suit all family members
- antihistamines if anyone in your family is known to be prone to allergy
- a small list of emergency procedures to help you cope if you are in a panic. (You could photocopy pages 28 to 48 of this book and keep them in your first aid box, so that you will always have the information to hand. Include useful telephone numbers such as doctor's surgery, hospital casualty and a taxi firm.)

Useful items:

❏ antiseptic ointment or lotion. Casualty departments often use sterile saline solution instead
   (If you have neither, clean a wound with water)
❏ a selection of plasters and dressings
❏ an eye bath
❏ a triangular sling
❏ a selection of bandages for different purposes,
   e.g. crepe for sprains and gauze for dressing
❏ clingwrap for burns. Chop a roll to a size to fit
   your first aid box and wrap it round the burned
   area like a bandage, leaving it slightly loose for
   the burned area to swell
❏ arnica cream for bruises (optional)
❏ tweezers for thorns
❏ specialist items if you have a patient with special
   needs among your friends and family, such as
   glucose for a diabetic.

Bites and stings

Dog and other animal bites

Always contact your surgery or local Accident and Emergency department (A&E) if there are cuts or lacerations, which may need stitching. If a hand or foot has been bitten, you will need to see a doctor to check there is no tendon or joint damage. Where the skin has not been broken or is simply punctured by a tooth you can deal with it yourself. Wash the area carefully and apply a plaster. A tetanus immunisation will normally only be required if a child has *not* had baby immunisations at 8, 12 and 16 weeks and a pre-school booster. (All children are offered a pre-school booster which includes tetanus immunisation. This covers them for a further ten years.) Keep an eye on bite areas for a day or two to check for infection – redness, swelling and tenderness.

Seek medical advice immediately for snake bites.

Insect stings

A wasp sting will not usually be left behind in the skin whereas a bee sting will. This can be removed by flicking or gently scraping with a fingernail or blunt knife. The area will be red and swollen.

The bite is usually painful for a few minutes and children will invariably be very upset.

Wasp and bee stings –
what you can do

❏ Remove a bee sting and apply some baking soda (sodium bicarbonate) powder mixed with a little water.

❏ For wasp stings use vinegar. If there is swelling, children over the age of two can have antihistamines (e.g. 5ml of Piriton syrup).

Contact the doctor for a sting if:

❏ the child has had a previous severe reaction to a sting

❏ the child is stung in the mouth

❏ the child later develops a temperature and the sting area is red, swollen and tender. This may mean the area has become infected.

If the child becomes breathless or there are other signs of allergy such as a blotchy rash or swelling, dial 999.

Bleeding

With cuts and other injuries which cause bleeding, there are two words to remember – *pressure* and *elevation*. You can stop virtually any bleeding by raising the affected part of the body above the level of the heart and applying pressure with a pad made out of cloth – a piece of clothing, a tea towel or similar. In any case of severe bleeding (haemorrhage) keep pressing firmly on the bleeding area until you can get help from a doctor or ambulance staff. Never apply a tourniquet.

Small cuts and grazes

Thoroughly clean the wound and apply a dressing such as a plaster or gauze pad. Continue to apply some pressure to stop the bleeding as long as there is no glass in the cut. A doctor should be consulted if there is the possibility of some foreign body in the cut. The face, scalp and hands have a very good blood supply so you may need to apply pressure there for 15 minutes or more.

Larger cuts

If you think the wound will need stitching, take the child to your nearest A&E unit or, in rural areas, to your doctor's surgery. A&E staff may use stitches, steristrips (paper stitches), staples or surgical glue. They will avoid stitching fingers if they think the injury will continue to swell, in which case the stitches would hamper the blood supply.

Puncture wounds

In cases where a large sharp object has punctured the skin, don't attempt to remove it. This will be done in hospital where severe bleeding can be properly treated.

Small objects, such as a pin or a thorn, can be safely removed.

Bruising and bumps

Most children will go through a phase of having permanently bruised knees or shins! Parents often discover these at bath time when it is generally too late to do anything about it. If you are presented with a bump soon after it has happened, gentle pressure and/or an ice pack (either ice cubes in a polythene bag placed in a tea towel or a packet of frozen peas in a tea towel) can reduce the swelling and subsequent bruising. If bruising occurs frequently without known injury make an appointment for the child to see your doctor.

Bumps on the head or face cause local swelling which may develop at an alarming rate into a bump which can be the size of a plum. This is frightening if you haven't seen it happen before. Check for head injury symptoms (see page 41) and apply an ice pack. The bump will slowly subside and leave a large bruise which will disappear over ten days or so.

Excessive bruising, and bruising after trivial injuries should be investigated, so make an appointment at your surgery.

Burns

Always treat a burn or scald with cold water. If possible, immerse the burned area in cold water for at least ten minutes, but avoid prolonged application over a large area. Remove any constricting clothing or jewellery before the injured area begins to swell. Never apply any creams or greases.

If hot liquid has spilt on to clothing remove the clothing. If you can't get it off immediately, wet it with cool or cold water, then try to remove it. You must act quickly to avoid severe burns. If hands are affected do the same, but then put the child's hand in a clean polythene bag while you contact the doctor. Apply clean wet wraps such as towels or even clingfilm to the burn while you transport the child to the surgery or A&E. Clingfilm is more effective than cold water after the initial period.

You should contact your doctor, practice nurse or hospital casualty department immediately for all but the most minor scalds.

Choking

If a child accidentally inhales something from the mouth choking will result. Coughing nearly always dislodges whatever is causing the obstruction to the air passages, but if this does not happen quickly then you will have to help to dislodge it.

Choking – what to do

❏ Look inside the mouth to see if it is possible to remove the object. Do not put your fingers into the back of the throat in case you push the object further down the windpipe.

Babies under one year

❏ Lie the baby along your forearm or thigh with the head facing down. Support the baby's head by holding the jaw.
❏ Give up to five firm slaps between the shoulder blades.

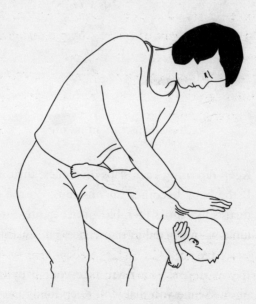

Back slaps in an infant

❏ If this does not work, rest the baby on your thigh with one arm supporting the back. Apply two fingers to an area a finger's width below the nipples in the middle of the chest and press down about 2cm.

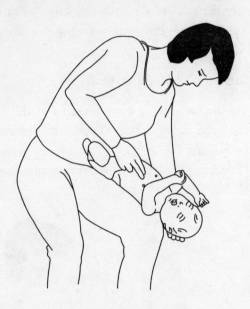

Chest thrusts in an infant

❏ Keep repeating back slaps then chest thrusts.
❏ If the baby becomes unconscious, do the chest thrusts five times then blow once gently into the lungs as instructed in the section on resuscitation (see page 45).
❏ If you are on your own, take your baby to the phone while you dial 999. Keep following these instructions until help arrives.

Children over one year

❏ Initially encourage your child to spontaneously cough up the obstruction.

❏ If this fails and your child starts gasping for breath then place him over your knee, with his head down, and apply up to five firm back slaps between the shoulder blades.

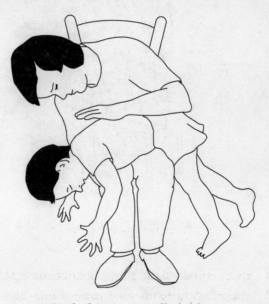

Back slaps in a small child

❏ If unsuccessful, apply chest thrusts. Place the heel of the hand two fingers' width in from the base of the breastbone and press five times.

❏ If the above procedures fail to dislodge the object, then try abdominal thrusts. **Do not attempt abdominal thrusts on infants under one year as they can damage internal organs.** To carry out this procedure on:

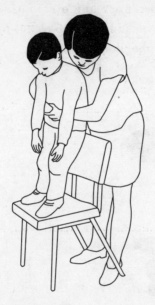

Abdominal thrusts in a standing child

a) *a conscious child*. Move behind the child and encircle them with your arms. It may be necessary to stand them on a chair if they're small. Form a fist with one hand placing the thumb side against the abdomen just above the navel. Grasp the fist with the other hand and perform a series of up to five quick upward thrusts, with each being a separate movement.

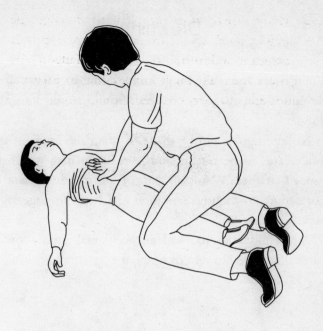

Abdominal thrusts with victim lying unconscious

b) *an unconscious child*. Place the child on his back. Using a tongue-jaw lift, open the airway and remove the object if visible. Attempt ventilation. If unsuccessful, kneel astride victim's hips. Place the heel of the hand on the abdomen just above the navel and place the other hand on top of the fist. Perform a series of up to five upward thrusts, with each being a separate movement.

❏ Note if your child stops breathing at any time you must start resuscitation (see page 45) and make sure an ambulance is called.

Drowning

When water enters the lungs it blocks the air passages and prevents the passage of oxygen from the air into the blood.

No attempt should be made to drain the lungs. If the child seems to be unconscious, breathing may well have stopped. If there is still no sign of life it is important to start mouth-to-mouth respiration and heart massage right away (see page 45).

Any child who has had an accidental immersion in water should be brought to hospital.

Electric shock

Mild electric shocks cause pain and the child will jump away from the source of the shock and be quite distressed. Many electric shocks are much more serious than this. At best they will cause burns and at worst cause the heart to stop beating.

Firstly, shut off the electricity supply at the socket or the mains before you touch the child. If the child is unconscious and not breathing, call an ambulance and start heart massage and mouth-to-mouth respiration (see page 45). If the child is still conscious check for burns. Electrical burns can be very deep and may be worse than they look. Treat as for burns (page 32) and attend A&E for all but the most trivial burns.

Eye injuries

If something has gone into a child's eye – whether it is sand, dust, soap or chemicals – wash the eye with water.

It needs to be done right away. Dust can be washed away with water and chemicals will be diluted, thereby reducing the risk of damage to the eye. Tilt the head sideways so that the affected eye is lowermost. Using a jug pour the water on to the inner corner of the eye and use your other hand to keep the eyelids open. If you can see a piece of grit or other foreign body, try to remove it with a cotton bud or a folded tissue. It is important that you do not try to remove anything that is embedded in the eye. If you are worried at all attend A&E or your doctor's surgery. Noting the name of any chemical involved may be helpful.

Take your child to the doctor or A&E if she has had a direct blow to the eye.

Fractures

'Fracture' means a broken bone. It is usually caused by trauma from an injury, although in the brittle bone disease *osteogenesis imperfecta* (see page 71) bones may be broken with minimal trauma. If you suspect that your child may have a fracture then you should attend A&E. Suspicious signs are inability to bear weight on the leg, ankle or foot;

marked swelling or tenderness over one site and deformity is also highly suspicious. A child who does not seem to be using one arm or hand after an injury may have a fracture. However, the ability to move fingers or toes after an injury does not rule out the presence of a fracture. Fractures of the bones of the wrist can be present in children without any swelling, bruising or deformity. In these cases there is little point in attending your surgery and you should go straight to A&E, where the doctor will assess the need for an x-ray.

The majority of childhood fractures need only manipulation (repositioning) and the application of a plaster cast, with no need for the skin to be breached.

Fractures of the fingers and toes are often treated by strapping them to the next finger or toe. This acts like a natural splint. The same happens in fractures of the long bones inside the hands and feet; the bones on either side can act as splints and so these often don't need plaster.

Skull fractures are rarely visible. **Serious head injury should be suspected if there is any abnormality of the conscious level, especially loss of consciousness, after a head injury or if there is persistent vomiting. Skull fracture may be present without these symptoms.**

Head injury

The rough and tumble of normal play can often lead to injury and head injury is common.

Head injury – contact your doctor if:

❏ the child is at all confused or cannot remember what happened
❏ there is abnormal behaviour
❏ the child has been unconscious or knocked out
❏ the child has vomited after the injury
❏ there is bleeding from the ear
❏ there is unusual drowsiness.

Bumps on the head can cause swelling to arise at an alarming rate. Apply a cold compress (i.e. a cloth rinsed out in cold water and squeezed dry). As long as the child is not showing any of the other signs listed above it is safe to wait and see. You will usually see the lump reduce in size and the child will usually return to normal in an hour or so.

Nosebleeds

Nosebleeds or *epistaxis* can occur at any age. They are more likely if the nose is congested by hay fever or a cold.

Nosebleeds – what you can do

❏ Pressure is the key word in any bleeding. For nosebleeding press just under the hard part of the bridge of the nose.

❏ Keep pressing for at least ten minutes. The bleeding will stop. Do not tip the head back.

❏ If it repeatedly starts again after releasing the pressure, contact your doctor for advice.

❏ Once the bleeding is stopped the child should be kept calm and avoid running around for the next hour or so.

Poisoning

Always contact your surgery or local A&E immediately if you suspect that your child has swallowed pills, medicine or household chemicals. Always check that missing pills haven't spilled on to the floor, but when you are sure, or even suspect, that your child has swallowed some do not delay in contacting your doctor or A&E – whichever is likely to be the quicker.

Do not attempt to make the child vomit. If your child loses consciousness you may have to start resuscitation. See page 45.

Your doctor may need to seek advice from the local poisons advice centre, so try to have as much information as possible available, e.g. number of tablets, the name of the chemical from the label and manufacturer. You may think that small quantities will probably do no harm but always seek advice first. Take the bottle with you.

Some household chemicals are easy for a child to reach and contain potentially dangerous substances. Recent changes mean that medicines which your pharmacist may once have put into a childproof bottle are now dispensed in easy to open blister packs.

To prevent such accidents, always keep medicines locked away. Never put household or garden chemicals in bottles which may attract children, such as lemonade bottles. As soon as they are old enough, educate your children about berries, toadstools etc. Families who use surma, the Asian cosmetic, should always make sure that they are using a lead-free surma.

The recovery position

If a child is lying on their back unconscious, kneel beside them and move them on to their side into the recovery position:

❏ Look in the mouth and clear away any vomit or other obvious obstruction. Be careful not to push an object in further. Gently tilt the casualty's head back to keep airway open.

❏ Straighten the limbs. Take the arm nearest to you and tuck it under the child's body. The open palm should be under the upper thigh.

❏ Bring the furthest arm towards you across the body, and hold the back of this hand against the child's cheek. Use your other hand to grasp the leg furthest and bend it at the knee, keeping the foot flat on the ground.

❏ Making sure that the child's hand remains on their cheek, pull the bent leg towards you and roll the victim onto their side. Ensure that they do not roll all the way over onto their stomach.

❏ The 'top' leg should remain bent, with the hip and knee at right angles to the body. Pull the underneath arm out behind the child to prevent him or her from rolling back. Ensure that the head is still resting on the child's hand and is tilted well back to keep the airway open.

Resuscitation

We can't say the following enough. Remember the ABC of resuscitation: Airway, Breathing, Circulation.

Airway

❑ When a child is found unconscious, the first thing to think about is the airway. Is it blocked?

❑ Look in the mouth and clear away any vomit or other obvious obstruction. Be careful not to push an object in further than it already is.

❑ Loosen tight clothing.

Breathing

❑ Check for breathing – listen at the mouth, look for the chest moving, and see if you can feel breath on your cheek. Try not to spend more than ten seconds on this.

❑ If the child is not breathing, tilt the chin backwards slightly.

❑ Take a deep breath, put your mouth over the mouth, pinch the nose and breathe into the lungs. With smaller children you will have to put your mouth over their mouth and nose.

❑ Repeat this around 20 times per minute – once every three seconds.

❑ Check for circulation after the first two inflations.

Circulation

❏ It can often be difficult to find a baby's pulse. The best place is on the inside of the upper arm, midway between the shoulder and elbow. Place two fingers over the inside of the arm and press in towards the bone. If no pulse is present start heart massage.

Heart massage

❏ Place the child on a firm surface.
❏ Using your fingertips in small children, or the heel of your hand in older children, apply pressure to the bottom of the breastbone about 2cm below the nipples.
❏ For a baby, apply pressure one finger's breadth below the nipples with two fingers.
❏ Try to press about once per second with older children and slightly faster with babies and toddlers – around 100 times per minute. Press down between 1cm and 2cm.
❏ If you are alone give one breath to every five chest compressions. If you have help give two breaths for every five chest compressions applied by your helper.
❏ If you are alone, try to call 999 or shout for help after one minute. Then quickly return to resuscitation.

❏ You should *always* get help. If you need to go to fetch someone, take the baby or toddler with you and continue resuscitation as you go.

❏ If the child regains consciousness before the ambulance arrives place her in the recovery position.

❏ Do not leave the child alone.

Sprains and strains

A sprain is a torn ligament. Ligaments are the tissues which hold our bones together. One of the commonest sprains is of the ligament that holds the fibula bone of the shin on to the heel bone. This is a sprained ankle.

Sprains are less common in children than in adults and if an under-5 is unable to walk because of injury, a fracture is more likely.

Sprains should be treated right away with pressure from a cold compress (i.e. a cloth rinsed out in cold water and squeezed dry). Later the joint should be rested and supported with a crepe or tubular bandage. If you are worried about the possibility of fracture you should attend A&E. Give paracetamol or apply a painkilling cream. Ask your pharmacist for advice.

A strain usually refers to a pulled muscle. This causes sudden pain over the muscle and there may be slight swelling. It is treated in the same way as a sprain.

Swallowed objects

Babies and toddlers love to put things in their mouths and not uncommonly end up swallowing them. Most coins and small toys will pass through the stomach and intestine and appear a few days later. Do consult the doctor, though.

Follow the instructions given above on choking if the object seems to be causing breathing difficulty. Follow the instructions on poisoning if the article is a pill or chemical. If the object is sharp or quite large always call your doctor for advice.

If a child swallows a battery, take her to A&E immediately because batteries contain corrosive substances.

6

A–Z of common ailments and how to treat them

In these entries, words that appear in **bold type** are the titles of other entries to which you should refer for more information.

Abdominal pain

When doctors talk about the abdomen they mean any part of the body between the lower edge of the ribcage and the groin.

Abdominal pain can occur in a wide range of illnesses, from infections such as gastro-enteritis, urine infections and diabetes to appendicitis. Pain can be constant or colicky, i.e. it comes in waves like labour contractions. Colic pain often goes away completely between waves. The pain associated with tummy bugs is often colicky and is due to spasms of the muscles of the intestines. Pain may also be associated with certain foods and the particular food may become obvious after two or three episodes.

In children there may be pain linked to diseases in other parts of the body such as tonsillitis or an ear infection. Children who suffer from sickle cell disease may get bouts of severe abdominal pain.

Appendicitis pain confuses many people. They know that it may move but don't know where. Essentially any organ in the abdomen which becomes inflamed may cause pain in the middle of the tummy. As the inflammation worsens the membrane which covers the organs, the peritoneum, becomes affected and the pain moves to the area of that organ – in the case of the appendix the right lower corner of the tummy. This is what is known as peritonitis. Most surgeons agree that appendices don't grumble and that recurrent abdominal pain is due to a cause such as constipation.

Parents usually guess that their baby has abdominal pain when the infant draws his knees up, goes red in the face and screams. This can happen when an infant has become constipated (see **constipation**) and also when a baby suffers from **colic**. However if there is blood or blood-stained mucus in the bowel motion or nappy then call the doctor immediately. This could be a sign of a potentially serious condition called intussusception in which the intestine folds back on itself, causing a blockage.

Abdominal pain is often a sign of an emotional upset such as bullying at school. This should always be suspected if a child often has tummy pain in the morning.

Children, especially younger children, may not have

the vocabulary to explain if they don't feel well and tummy pain is simply their way of communicating that things are not right.

What you can do

If your child is old enough to tell you that his tummy hurts, he will probably be able to explain where it hurts. Have other members of the family had diarrhoea or have there been some cases at nursery? Does he complain when he passes urine? Does the urine have a strong smell and is it cloudy or even blood stained? Does his breath smell different? Is he constipated?

Try paracetamol at the recommended dose for the child's age. Paracetamol will not mask the symptoms of more serious problems such as appendicitis but will often help the pain associated with, for example, diarrhoea or tonsillitis.

A hot water bottle (not too hot, of course!) can be soothing if placed on the tummy.

If pain seems severe and has not been helped by paracetamol, call the doctor for advice. For recurrent, less severe pain make an appointment at the surgery. If there is the possibility of collecting some urine for the doctor to test, do so.

Abscess or boil

An abscess is a collection of pus and is most usual under the skin where, for example, a hair has been pulled out and infection has got into the hair follicle. An abscess is a tender red swelling sometimes with a yellow 'head'. One occurring in the fold next to a fingernail or toenail is called a whitlow. Small abscesses will often get better by themselves and some will burst themselves with or without the help of a poultice – a paste applied to the skin which helps to draw the infection out. Larger ones may need an antibiotic or lancing, which means that the pus is drained. For very large abscesses this may be done under a general anaesthetic, while smaller ones may be incised with a freezing liquid which is sprayed onto the surface just before the abscess is lanced. Don't be tempted to lance abscesses by yourself, even with a clean needle. See your GP or your practice nurse.

Tooth abscesses need to be dealt with by a dentist. Your GP is likely to have had no dentistry training at all and would not have the facilities in their surgery to diagnose a tooth abscess unless it is really obvious. This means that most GPs will be reluctant to treat dental abscesses unless a dentist has made the diagnosis. All children should be registered with an NHS dentist and this will entitle them to have 24-hour access to dental advice and treatment if your dentist feels it can't wait until the next day.

Adenoids

The adenoids play a part in the body's defence against infection. They lie at the bottom of the Eustachian tubes which connect the internal part of the ear with the back of the throat. They cannot be seen from the mouth. Indications that they might be enlarged include snoring and frequent ear infections especially if this results in **glue ear**. In this case an ear, nose and throat specialist might advise removal of the adenoids. This is a straightforward operation. Between the ages of one and eight years, infections of the tonsils and adenoids are very common following colds. After this age these tissues often start to shrink and infections become less common. This is one of the reasons for the reluctance of doctors to refer older children to a specialist. A few unlucky people will continue to have tonsillitis and ear infections throughout their teens and into their twenties.

Allergies

Anyone, including children, can develop allergies to just about anything. Symptoms include a rash, itch, swelling, breathing difficulty, sneezing and watery eyes. Those who are severely allergic to such things as bee stings may collapse and become seriously ill (which is called anaphylaxis). It is rare in young children and is more likely if there has been a previous reaction to a substance.

Recently there have been worries about the apparent increase in the incidence of people allergic to nuts and nut products. Peanut (groundnut) oil is used as the main fat in many cakes, biscuits and other foods. Manufacturers of such products may use the same equipment to produce food which does not contain nuts and as a result it may be contaminated by nuts. In these circumstances manufacturers warn consumers by stating on the packaging that their product may contain traces of nuts. Those allergic to nuts – and, indeed, any other substance that may occur in processed food – must be very cautious about what they eat.

What you can do

Allergies may be caused by things we eat, things we put on our skin or things we breathe. Minor reactions may need no treatment other than to stop using the allergen (whatever it is that causes the allergy), e.g. washing powder.

Urticaria is a rash which is linked to allergies. It very often comes on soon after the person has eaten something they are allergic to. It can start by looking like nettle stings – small raised white spots with a red area around them. It progresses by spreading outwards to form raised patches which can literally expand as you watch them. They are often intensely itchy. If the reaction is localised to one area of the body, does not appear to be spreading and is not linked to swelling of the face, then it is safe to apply calamine lotion, give some antihistamine such as chlorpheniramine (Piriton syrup – not to be given to children under one year) and wait and see. In the more severe reactions, where you can see that the rash is developing, you should take the child to your surgery or A&E immediately. Swelling of the face is most obvious around the eyes. They appear puffy and may look as if they are closing. Swelling of the face may be followed by difficulty in breathing so don't delay in seeking help.

Less severe reactions can be treated with antihistamines. Your pharmacist will advise you but will usually recommend that children under the age of six see their GP first.

People who know they are allergic (e.g. to bee stings or nuts) can carry a special injection kit containing adrenaline with them to be given in case of anaphylaxis. This is available for children as well as adults.

New advice has been published on the subject of nut allergy. We are not certain why so many people are becoming allergic to nuts, but there is a possibility of sensitisation during pregnancy and breastfeeding. Therefore women who are pregnant or breastfeeding and who have a family history of allergy are advised to abstain from nuts. It is not recommended at the moment that all women avoid nuts.

Anaemia

See **blood disorders**.

Anal fissure

A fissure is a small crack in the back passage which usually results from an episode of constipation. It is often extremely painful and may result in the child deliberately avoiding emptying the bowels because of the pain. Obviously this creates a vicious circle with further constipation.

Treatment involves using medicine to soften the bowel motion plus painkilling ointment to apply to the back passage if needed. It is not recommended that very young children have bran or other similar fibre but roughage can be given in the form of fruit and vegetables, and for all ages it is a good idea to increase the intake of water to keep the stool soft.

Antibiotics

Antibiotics are drugs which fight infection. Doctors generally restrict the term to those that kill bacteria. Examples of bacterial infections include pneumonia and tonsillitis. The vast majority of winter ailments – such as colds, flu and chest infections – are caused by a different type of organism called a virus. These do not respond to antibiotics.

When penicillin was first discovered it was effective against a wide range of bacteria. As its use increased, bacteria were able to 'learn' to combat the antibiotic and it is now effective against only a limited number of them. Research has produced dozens of new antibiotics since then but many have suffered the same fate. Doctors are becoming increasingly concerned about escalating resistance to antibiotics and many now feel that we should avoid using them at all for mild infections. They certainly should not be used for conditions that are known to be viral.

Particularly worrying is the emergence of highly resistant bacteria. These have been nicknamed 'superbugs'.

Even the most powerful antibiotics reserved for hospital use fail to kill some of these bacteria.

We have few effective treatments for viral illnesses. This means that diseases such as flu, colds and most sore throats need to be treated symptomatically (with drugs such as paracetamol for fever and antihistamines for stuffy noses and catarrh). Most people can self-diagnose a cold but any unexpected or worrying symptoms should be reported to a doctor. The doctor would then be able to decide whether to advise over-the-counter remedies or issue a prescription.

Appendicitis

See **abdominal pain**.

Asthma

The definition of asthma is a reversible narrowing of the air passages in the lungs. This causes wheeze (a whistling sound heard as the child breathes out) and, in younger children, a cough which is often more noticeable at night or after the child has been running around. The narrowing of the air passages is caused by inflammation in the lining of the passages, which in turn is caused by exposure to certain stimuli. These stimuli may differ from person to person. Common causes are dust from the coats of pets, cold air, infections and house dust mites – which are present all over the house, especially in mattresses, pillows etc.

One in five children in the UK now uses an inhaler at some time. Babies who have been breastfed for at least three months are less likely to suffer from wheeze than bottle-fed infants, as are babies who have not been given solid food until 15 weeks of age. These benefits last throughout early childhood.

Many parents are dismayed when a diagnosis of asthma is made. They fear that their child may be weak and unable to take part in sports or other activities. Happily, since the advent of effective therapy the vast majority of asthmatic children grow up to live normal lives. Asthma does need to be monitored, however, and most surgeries will offer regular check-ups. The commonest test used to monitor asthma is the peak expiratory flow rate. This is a measurement of the amount of air which can be blown out of the lung's air passages in a set amount of time. Air passages which are narrowed by inflammation will not be able to blow air out as fast as normal-size air passages. The device used to check this measurement is called a peak flow meter and these are calibrated to measure the air in litres per minute. The doctor or nurse will ask the child to breathe into the machine quite sharply. The level expected varies according to the child's height. During an asthma attack the level falls and the treatment given will depend on how much it falls. These devices can be kept at home. They are simple to use and to read and can help parents to judge how wheezy a child is and therefore when to seek help from a doctor.

Nebulisers are devices which use moistened air to help deliver a drug into the lungs. The drugs given through a nebuliser are exactly the same as those in inhalers although the dose may be bigger. Parents of asthmatic children sometimes ask whether they should consider buying one of these. They are not usually available from the NHS although they can sometimes be borrowed for a few days during an attack. While it is true that a small number of children may benefit from having one at home, for the vast majority of asthmatics a spacer device is just as good. These are made of plastic, they may be balloon shaped and they are available on prescription. They allow young children to use aerosol inhalers easily and can be helpful to asthmatics of all ages during an attack. When they are used there is less worry about getting the technique of inhalation absolutely right. They are cumbersome, however, and many children will use an inhaler on its own for day-to-day use. Spacers should be washed once a week in soapy water and dried on the draining board, not with a tea towel.

Doctors seldom make the diagnosis of asthma from one episode of wheeze. Your doctor will look at the overall pattern of illnesses in each individual child. Episodes of wheeze should be documented in the child's records and therefore the child should be taken to the surgery when they occur.

Asthma is treated by:

- ❏ airway relaxer drugs given by inhaler (or syrup in young children) when wheeze is present
- ❏ prevention drugs, also given by inhaler, taken regularly every day. Older children can usually be taught to manage their inhaler use by themselves and will often need to take an inhaler to school. It is important that school staff allow the child to have the inhaler with them especially when playing sport. Each type of inhaler has a known number of 'puffs'. Some even have the individual doses numbered so it is easy to check how many have been taken
- ❏ in severe attacks of wheeze doctors may prescribe oral steroid drugs, even for very young children. Steroids are one of the most powerful treatments available for inflammation. Side effects are fairly rare if the steroid course is kept short
- ❏ oral medication which can be given in medicine, tablet and capsule form for both treatment and prevention of asthma.

Asthma – general advice

- ❏ Try not to expose children to cigarette smoke.
- ❏ Attend asthma clinics as often as your doctor recommends.
- ❏ Learn as much as you can about the condition so you understand the illness and its treatment.
- ❏ If a child becomes very breathless contact your doctor without delay.

Athlete's foot

Athlete's foot is a fungal infection of the skin between the toes, sometimes spreading over the sole of the foot. It causes flaking and cracking of the skin and is often itchy.

Athlete's foot – what you can do

- ❏ Fresh air is the easiest cure. Therefore avoid letting your child wear trainers all day.
- ❏ Opt for cotton socks, which absorb sweat.
- ❏ Always dry toes well after baths and swimming.
- ❏ Use an anti-fungal cream such as clotrimazole. There are also anti-fungal powders and sprays.

Autism

Autism is a disorder which affects a child's behaviour. The child is unable to relate to others in the normal way. The child may seem distant and not responsive to affection. These children often spend hours playing by themselves and display repetitive behaviour. The child may become quite distressed if prevented from carrying out ritualistic behaviour such as doing things in a certain order. All children derive a sense of security from routines but in autism routine becomes obsessional.

There is no cure for autism but some behavioural therapy has been shown to be helpful. Children should be referred to a specialist as soon as the condition is suspected.

Bedwetting

One in ten children still wet the bed regularly at the age of five and one in twenty still do at the age of ten.

Children learn bladder control at different ages so don't compare your own child with others. By all means try the potty or toilet trainer seat but don't force it if the child is not ready. Achievement of bladder control may be hindered by such things as urine infections or emotional problems. If you suspect an infection because the urine smells foul or the child is wetting during the day as well, ask your practice nurse for a bottle to collect a specimen for the laboratory (or an adhesive bag for very young children).

If infection has been excluded and the child is under five then be patient! Bladder control is very likely to come of its own accord. Give praise when there is a dry bed but try to stay calm when the bed is wet. Older children can use star charts, alarms and medication available on prescription to help them achieve control. If you have any concerns about potty training, bladder control or bedwetting, contact your health visitor.

Behavioural problems

This is difficult to define as what may be one person's behavioural problem may be another's creative expression. In general, though, most parents will encounter from time to time forms of behaviour in their children which they find difficult to cope with, and which they may regard as anti-social. Children do need to learn appropriate behaviour as they grow, but at the same time parents need to understand that just as Rome wasn't built in a day so children learn bit by bit. For example, most two-year-olds do not take easily to sharing toys and this has resulted in many a toddler group bust-up. The same children at the age of four may have realised that sharing can actually be fun. It therefore doesn't make sense to upset toddlers by trying to force them to share and it is better to try to distract one of them to play with something else. This is not pandering to them – it is simply exploitation of the natural course of events.

It is up to each family to set their own ground rules

and to be as strict as they choose to be. In general, it is a good idea to be consistent. Children will happily play one adult off another if they think that it might result in them getting their own way! And never make threats which you can't carry out. Children have amazingly good memories and won't be fooled twice.

If you feel that your child's behaviour is becoming a problem take some time to think it through. Is it a problem just in your eyes or are other people finding it difficult too? Could it just be a phase that will pass and is therefore best ignored in the short term, or are you expecting too much for the age of your child? Are you being inconsistent and giving mixed messages to your child? It is important to remember to praise, and sometimes reward, the behaviour that you want so that your child receives positive messages from you.

Never forget that children can be affected by stress as much as adults and this may manifest itself as 'bad' behaviour. If there are changes in the household such as a house move or a new brother or sister, changes in routine such as going to nursery or even arguments in the family, then you should anticipate changes in your child's behaviour. Try to not get upset yourself if she seems to be much naughtier than usual. Talk to your health visitor.

Birthmarks

So-called 'stork marks' are very common. These consist of a triangular red mark on the forehead and another red mark at the back of the neck. They will fade over a few months and do not need treatment.

Strawberry naevi (birthmarks) may increase in size over the first year or two but will then gradually shrink. They will have shrunk markedly by the time the child is seven years old. Parents are often alarmed by these as they can be a considerable size and can be raised from the skin. However, unless they are causing secondary problems such as pressure on other tissues (e.g. in the neck) it is better to wait for them to resolve on their own.

Port-wine stains (a deep red colour) do not fade and, depending on the site and the size, may be amenable to plastic surgery or laser treatment. These are flat.

In babies with dark skin there may be a pigmented area at the bottom of the back. This has the appearance of a bruise and is called a blue spot. Most will fade in time but may take up to two years.

Babies may also have brown birthmarks like moles. These can vary in size from a millimetre or two to a centimetre or more. They may also be hairy. These are harmless and do not disappear.

Bladder infections

See **kidney infections**.

Blood disorders

The blood contains cells which perform different functions. Red cells carry oxygen from the lungs to all the tissues of the body. White cells fight infection and are involved in allergic reactions. Platelets help the blood to clot when blood vessels are injured and there is bleeding. The bone marrow produces these cells.

Anaemia

The chemical responsible for transporting oxygen is called haemoglobin and a lack of haemoglobin is called anaemia. This can arise if there is insufficient iron or folic acid in the diet or if there is bleeding. Anaemia also occurs in some chronic illnesses such as colitis and some types of arthritis. Anaemia causes tiredness, breathlessness and dizziness. It is relatively rare in children although it may be seen in children who do not eat a balanced diet. Most of our iron comes from meat, fish and eggs. Vegetarians are only at more risk of anaemia if their diet is not well balanced. Girls who suffer from heavy periods may become anaemic if their diet does not contain iron-rich foods. Premature babies are also at risk of anaemia. Anaemia is diagnosed with a blood test and treated with iron or folic acid, depending on which is in short supply.

In thalassaemia, the haemoglobin is not normal. Children who suffer from this condition are anaemic and may not grow properly. This condition is inherited and more common in children of Middle Eastern origin.

Anaemia also occurs in conditions where the blood cells are broken more quickly than they are replaced. Cell breakdown is called haemolysis, so these anaemias are called haemolytic anaemias; the main types are thalassaemia and **sickle cell disease**.

Haemolytic disease of the newborn

This condition may result when a Rhesus negative mother carries a Rhesus positive child. This could happen if the baby's father is Rhesus positive. The Rhesus title refers to a chemical on the red blood cells. If there is any contact between the mother's blood and the baby's during the pregnancy the mother may 'reject' the baby's blood by producing antibodies against it. This results in haemolysis. It is potentially very serious and the reaction may become worse in subsequent pregnancies. This is why it is important to know an expectant mother's blood group, even if she has suffered a miscarriage early in pregnancy. An injection of anti-D immunoglobulin can be given to Rhesus negative mothers to prevent this reaction from happening in the future.

Haemophilia

As well as platelets, we need a group of chemicals that interact with each other to clot blood. These are known as the clotting factors. A lack of any one of them will lead to a tendency to bruise and bleed. Haemophilia results from a deficiency of Factor Eight (or Factor VIII) which helps blood to coagulate. If this trait is carried on one of the sex chromosomes, sons of a female carrier may be affected. Children with this condition bleed after what appears to be a trivial injury and internal bleeding into joints or soft tissues may also occur. Factor Eight is available to administer to sufferers. Parents have to teach children affected how to avoid accidents which lead to bleeding and bruising.

Henoch-Schonlein purpura

There is a condition called Henoch–Schonlein purpura which results in minute red spots called petechiae, mainly on the backs of the legs. This occasionally happens after a sore throat and children may also have joint pains or abdominal pain. It is not usually serious but children are sometimes admitted to hospital for observation. The platelet count is not reduced greatly, if at all.

Idiopathic thrombocytopaenic purpura

Another condition which can affect children is idiopathic thrombocytopaenic purpura (purpura = bruising, thrombo–cytopaenic = not enough platelets, idiopathic = cause unknown). In this condition the platelet count is low, resulting in bruising, but the outcome is good and most children make a full recovery.

Leukaemia

Leukaemia is a form of cancer affecting the white blood cells. The cells produced do not function properly. Children with leukaemia have poor resistance to infection and may also be severely anaemic. They may also have a lack of platelets, so bruising or bleeding may occur.

There are different forms of leukaemia, some more aggressive than others, but most are treated with chemotherapy or radiotherapy. Chemotherapy consists of special drugs which kill cancer cells. Unfortunately most chemotherapy drugs also kill some normal cells. The ones most likely to be affected are those which naturally divide rapidly in the body, such as the lining of the intestine and the hair follicles. This is why people who have chemotherapy often suffer from diarrhoea and lose their hair. After a course of chemotherapy, these cells usually recover and start to work properly again.

Leukaemia remains a very serious illness in most children. Bone marrow transplants may be carried out if a suitable donor can be found.

Vitamin K

In newborn babies there may be a deficiency in clotting factors. This is particularly likely in pre-term babies, babies born by forceps or caesarean section and babies whose mothers take certain drugs such as anti-convulsive drugs. In the majority of babies this does not lead to any problems but in a few there may be internal bleeding. Vitamin K helps to prevent this and is therefore offered for all newborn babies.

In the early 1990s two research studies suggested that there may be a link between injected vitamin K and childhood **cancer**. Further research has been done since then and an increased risk of cancer has not been proven. Oral vitamin K is however available. A single oral dose is not totally effective in preventing haemorrhagic disease in breastfed babies and in those at higher risk; therefore further doses are advised if injected vitamin K is not wanted.

Bone disorders

Osteochondritis

Osteochondritis is a condition affecting the growing part of the bone. As children grow, the growing part or epiphysis adds on new bone. For example, the epiphyses of the long bones in the arms and legs are at the ends of the bones. When the child is fully grown the epiphysis joins up with the main part of the bone and the bone stops growing. Some 'growing pains' can be put down to osteochondritis. When the child has stopped growing the pains go away.

There is no specific treatment for osteochondritis unless it affects the part of the bone which faces into the joint (the articular surface). If pains become quite marked, resting the joint affected will help as will paracetamol or the junior version of ibuprofen. Thankfully, this condition does not usually result in long-term problems. The commonest joints affected are the hips (Perthe's disease), knees (Osgood–Schlatter's disease), spine (Scheuermann's disease), heel (Sever's disease) and foot (Kohler's disease).

In Perthe's disease, the child is most likely to be affected between the ages of five and nine, and may develop a limp and complain of pain in the hip. In this case doctors may try to immobilise the hip with a splint. Like the others, it usually goes away without leaving any problems.

Osteogenesis imperfecta

This is brittle bone disease, which causes fractures in children because the microscopic structure of the bone is defective. The fractures occur with the least trauma and until the disease has been diagnosed it has been known for parents to be suspected of deliberately harming their child. It is an inherited disorder and there is no specific treatment other than the prevention of the accidents which lead to the fractures.

Osteomyelitis

This is an infection of the bone which can occur after a fracture or injury. It can also be spread in the bloodstream to a bone from another source of infection in the body. It will usually result in a high temperature and tenderness in the affected bone. Osteomyelitis is rare and children suspected of having this infection will be admitted to hospital for treatment under the care of an orthopaedic consultant.

Breast enlargement

A degree of breast enlargement is normal in newborn babies due to stimulation by the mother's female hormones before birth. It happens in both girls and boys and does not need treatment.

Breath holding

When some children become acutely upset or angry they may hold their breath for what seems an unnaturally long time. You may find it happens more often if the child has been unwell or simply if they have had an active day and are very tired. It can be part of a tantrum and a sign of sheer frustration. The child's body may become very stiff and tense and his face red or even purple. Most children will eventually cry. If they don't, the attack may end with a loss of consciousness which will last for a few seconds or at the most up to a minute. This is extremely frightening but attacks end by themselves and no harm comes to the child. If worried consult your health visitor.

Breath holding – what you can do

❏ The first time it happens you will probably be too shocked to act quickly, but always try to remain calm. Once you have seen an attack you may be able to predict the next one by the pattern of the child's behaviour.

❏ Give him a gentle shake, holding his arms to get his attention, or blow onto his face to try to stop the attack in its tracks. Then give him a firm cuddle.

❏ After the second or third attack you will probably be quite adept at predicting attacks.

Breathlessness

Breathlessness can be caused by such things as infections, **asthma** or inhalation of a foreign body such as a peanut. (See also **asthma**, **bronchiolitis** and **croup**.) If it has started suddenly or the child's lips are blue you will need to take action.

Breathlessness – what to do

- ❑ Contact the doctor immediately –
- ❑ If breathing is rapid and/or shallow and the breathlessness is occurring at rest and a doctor cannot be contacted, take the child to an A&E unit (preferably in a hospital with a children's department) or dial 999 for an ambulance.

Children may become a bit more breathless than usual with a cough or cold. Noisy breathing can occur with a cough or cold and may simply be due to mucus in the nose or at the back of the throat. Babies and small children cannot effectively clear their throats or blow their noses as we do, but the mucus is not usually a problem. However, noisy breathing along with breathlessness will often need a doctor's advice. With a cold, the breathing rate is not usually much faster than normal unless the child has been exercising. Young children do not fake breathlessness so always take it seriously.

Bronchiolitis

Bronchiolitis is a viral infection which affects babies and young children. It causes fast, shallow breathing and a high temperature. It can cause wheeze. It is not normally treatable by antibiotics although a doctor may prescribe antibiotics if a secondary infection is suspected (see **viruses**).

If there is breathing difficulty the child may have to go to hospital.

If your baby or young child has rapid, shallow breathing, seek advice from a doctor immediately.

Cancer

All of the body's tissues and organs are made up of microscopic building blocks called cells. The cells of different organs have different characteristics. A trained person looking at a microscope slide can identify, by looking at the cells, which part of the body the tissue came from. Cells increase in number by dividing. Cells from different tissues also behave differently, some divide in two slowly and others quickly.

The main feature of cancer cells is that they have lost the ability to behave in the same way as normal cells. They also change in appearance and this can be seen with a microscope. They tend to divide more quickly than the normal cells around them. The extent to which this causes problems depends on the organ involved, the amount of the organ which has been affected by the abnormal cells and the aggressiveness of the cancer cells, i.e. whether they divide quickly or slowly.

Cells may spread to other tissues and organs in the body, sometimes at a distance from the original cancer. This happens when the cells are malignant. Benign cells tend to stay as a group in the original organ, although they may still grow to an enormous size and cause symptoms. In general malignant cancers are more serious than benign.

The word 'tumour' is used to encompass both benign and malignant cancers. Doctors tend to use 'cancer' for those which are malignant.

Childhood tumours are rare. They are also likely to be different from those that affect adults. Cancers such as breast or lung are exceptionally rare. The majority of childhood cancers arise in the bone marrow/lymphatic system, the brain and nervous system or the bone.

Malignant tumours are likely to be treated with chemotherapy or radiotherapy. They may also need surgical removal. Chemotherapy may be given by mouth or injected into the bloodstream. It consists of drugs which slow down or stop cell division. Unfortunately it cannot distinguish normal from abnormal and so those cells which naturally divide quickly in the body may be affected, in particular the hair and the lining of the intestine. Both chemotherapy and radiotherapy will be administered by specialist doctors.

Many benign tumours will be cured immediately after they are removed surgically.

See also 'leukaemia' under **blood disorders**.

Cerebral palsy

Cerebral palsy results from damage to the parts of the brain which control the body's movements and posture. This damage may occur before birth, during birth or during the first two years of life. The amount of damage caused may be slight or severe. The developing brain may be damaged by lack of oxygen, infections in the mother during pregnancy or a placenta which is not functioning properly. In many cases doctors are unable to find the exact cause. The blood vessels in the brain of premature babies are very fragile and are relatively easily damaged during labour and in the first few weeks of life, depending on the degree of prematurity. It follows that cerebral palsy is more common in very premature babies.

The damage may not always be evident at birth but become obvious as the baby grows. Some of the tests done at the eight-week screen check for cerebral palsy. If parents are worried that their baby has not reached any of the developmental milestones they should seek reassurance from their GP.

Children with cerebral palsy may need ongoing treatment throughout their childhood. Parents should always be involved in the treatment programme and in most cases will be able to help with exercises at home. Some sufferers from cerebral palsy may also have a mental handicap as a result of brain damage, but equally there may be no mental handicap whatsoever.

Chest infections

A chest infection often follows a cold. Most are what doctors would call an acute bronchitis. Don't confuse this with the chronic (long-standing) bronchitis that affects smokers. In an otherwise healthy child acute bronchitis will last around a week, cause a cough with or without phlegm and will gradually get better. The lungs have their own clearing mechanism and in a chest infection it is normal to have phlegm at the back of the throat in the morning. Coughing helps to clear the phlegm. These infections do not usually need treatment with antibiotics.

Pneumonia is more serious. The child will often have a very high temperature, perhaps with severe shivering, and be generally very unwell. It responds very well to antibiotics.

See also **bronchiolitis**.

Chest infections – what you can do

❑ If your child has had a cold which has 'gone onto her chest' but is otherwise well in herself (i.e. eating, playing etc.), it is worth waiting to see if she improves over 2–3 days. You can give a cough linctus at bedtime but avoid expectorants. Expectorants thin the mucus so that it is coughed up more easily, but will not make sleeping easy. Your pharmacist will advise you.

❑ If your child has a high temperature follow the instructions in the section on fever (page 2). If she still seems very unwell you should contact the doctor for advice.

❑ See also **cough**.

Chickenpox

See **childhood fevers**.

Chilblains

See **itch**.

Childhood fevers

Nearly all of the childhood fevers are caused by viruses and have no specific treatment. Always treat the fever with paracetamol and sponging (see Fevers, page 2). Treat itchy rashes such as chickenpox with calamine lotion or sponge with a solution of sodium bicarbonate (baking soda) in water applied with cotton wool.

The incubation period is the time from when the disease is first contracted by the child until the time when the first symptoms, usually fever, appear. Even when the diagnosis is obvious (e.g. if you have nursed a child with chickenpox before and know the signs), the surgery should be notified. Public health departments keep a check on the incidence of many infectious illnesses in communities and your surgery should notify them of all cases.

The following table summarises the significant features of common childhood fevers.

Illness	Incubation period	Exclusion period	Clinical features
Chickenpox	13–21 days	5 days from onset of rash; avoid contact with women in first 4 months of pregnancy.	Crops of blisters on the trunk
Erythema infectiosum (also known as fifth disease and slapped-cheek syndrome)	7–14 days	Nil	Mild illness 'Slapped cheek' appearance
German measles – see rubella			
Hand, foot and mouth disease	3–5 days	None	Spots on the hands, feet and roof of mouth (also on backs of legs and buttocks)
Measles	8–13 days	A few days before the rash appears until 5 days after it goes	Fever, catarrh, initially like very bad cold; rash appears on 3rd or 4th day, becoming widespread over the body; children often very unwell

Mumps	14–21 days	Five days from onset of swollen glands	Large, swollen glands under chin and in cheek, sometimes on one side only
Roseola infantum	10 days	Nil	High temperature at first; as fever subsides over 1–3 days a fine spreading rash appears, this is short-lasting
Rubella	14–21 days	7 days before the rash until 5 days after it appeared	Usually a mild illness with a fine rash more obvious after a bath
Scarlet fever (caused by bacteria, needs treatment with antibiotics)	2–5 days	5 days from commencing antibiotics	Tonsillitis, rash over trunk and face, tongue described as 'strawberry tongue'; skin, especially of fingers, may peel
Whooping cough (treated with antibiotics, child remains infectious until after 7 days' treatment)	7–10 days	Up to 3 weeks after fits of coughing start	Fever, catarrh followed by bouts of coughing, with or without a 'whoop', can go on for weeks

All pregnant women are offered a test for immunity to rubella. Because of the devastating effects on a fetus in early pregnancy, if there is any doubt about immunity keep an infectious child away from a woman in early pregnancy. Where there has been a risk of exposure blood tests can confirm whether the disease has been contracted.

Cleft palate

Cleft palate and hare lip are linked conditions. The palate forms in the fetus in two parts which eventually fuse together. If any part of this fusion fails, then a cleft palate or hare lip is the result. A hare lip is an obvious gap in the middle of the upper lip. A cleft palate is obvious only if you look inside the baby's mouth, when you will see the gap in the roof of the mouth. Either can interfere with feeding. The action of sucking requires the baby to move the tongue along the palate and if there is a gap then this action is hampered. Special teats are available for formula-fed babies to make feeding easier. Plastic surgery is available for these children.

Club foot

This is also known as *talipes*. It is caused by the feet being held in a fixed position in the womb so that the position is maintained after birth. It is more likely if the baby has been lying in the breech position. Talipes refers to a foot which curves inwards or outwards. The doctor who checks your baby after birth will check for talipes. In most cases the foot can be manipulated into the correct position and no treatment or only very simple treatment is required. In the more severe cases an operation may be needed.

Coeliac disease

Coeliac disease affects around 1 in 300 of the UK population. It is also called gluten enteropathy. This name refers to the fact that the intestine is adversely affected by gluten, a protein found in wheat. The intestine becomes 'flattened' and does not absorb food properly. The child may have chronic diarrhoea or loose stools. The stools may be pale, fatty and difficult to flush away. The child does not gain weight as expected. It is recommended that babies do not receive gluten in their diet until they are at least six months old and preferably not until 12 months of age. It is thought that the infant gut is too immature to cope with gluten.

The diagnosis is made by a blood test or a bowel biopsy. Once diagnosed, a child will have to exclude gluten from his diet. This means avoiding any food which is made from flour. Thankfully there is a huge range of gluten-free foods and some can be obtained on a prescription from your GP. They include flour, bread, pasta and biscuits. When gluten is excluded from the diet the bowel motions will return to normal and the child will gain weight. The sensitivity to gluten may remain for life. At the moment prescriptions for gluten-free foods are free.

If you decide to wean your baby on to commercially produced baby food, look for the 'ear of wheat' sign on the packet or jar which indicates that the product is gluten free.

Colds

The common cold is caused by viruses which are passed from person to person, often by coughing and sneezing. The incubation period is short – just a few days. There is usually fever, a sore throat and muscle aches and pains which move from one part of the body to another. This may be followed by a cough with phlegm which lasts for a few days or an ear infection. Colds may also sometimes be complicated by a **chest infection**, sinusitis or an **ear infection**. This explains why a cold may go on for longer than just a few days.

The average person will suffer up to five colds per year and these are more likely to occur in the winter time. There is not much that can be done to prevent a cold as they are so infectious. It used to be thought that vitamin C prevented colds. Although this could not be proven by medical research many people, including doctors, continue to take vitamin C in the winter. You will find that a child who has just started nursery or a new school will seem to suffer from one cold after another for a month or two and the rest of the family will follow suit.

Colds – what you can do

❏ See the section on Fevers (page 2) and follow the instructions. Antibiotics do not help colds or runny noses.
❏ Contact the doctor if
  – the child is unduly listless; remember that fever causes listlessness so always try para-cetamol
  – breathing is very fast or there is wheeze
  – the child develops a cough without having had a cold or the cough goes on after the cold symptoms have gone
  – there are signs from the checklist on **meningitis** on page 140.

Cold sores

Cold sores are caused by a virus and appear as sore spots around the mouth. They will often appear repeatedly in the same place. The virus can be passed to another person by contact, so avoid kissing your child if she has an active cold sore. You can buy an anti-viral cream from the chemist which should be applied frequently as soon as you are aware that a cold sore is starting. This may help to diminish the frequency and severity of future attacks but will not heal the current cold sore.

Colic

See also **abdominal pain**. Many babies seem to suffer from colicky pain during the first few months of life. This is often worse in the evening and causes them to cry relentlessly and draw their legs up.

The crying can be intermittent and the baby may seem to be settling between episodes. Parents should try to help the baby bring up wind by sitting him on their knee and gently rubbing his back. Gripe water may also help, as may carrying the baby in a sling. A mixture is available from your GP to be given with feeds. This is not helpful in every case and should only be continued if it *is* found to be helpful. After the age of three months episodes become less frequent and less severe; it is thought that colic is due to the immaturity of the gut in babies.

Complementary therapies

Many parents are concerned about side effects of drug treatment for illness and ask about other methods of treatment for themselves and their children. Probably the most commonly requested alternative therapy is homoeopathy. Homoeopathy involves using tiny doses of remedies which are mainly derived from plants. In many areas of the country you can see a GP who is also a fully qualified homoeopath through the NHS. Prescriptions may therefore be free of charge for children. To find such a GP you should contact your local Family Health Services Authority or in Scotland your Health Board.

Congenital abnormalities

Congenital means 'present at birth'. Abnormalities include hereditary conditions, conditions arising when the baby is growing in the womb and those arising through complications in labour.

Congenital dislocation of the hip

If a joint is dislocated, one of the bones is out of place. In the case of the hip, which is a ball and socket joint, the 'ball' (i.e. the head of the femur or thigh bone) is wholly or partially out of its socket, which is part of the pelvis.

Babies are checked at birth and at the eight-week screen for dislocation of the hip. This condition, if missed, can cause problems with walking in later life. If a hip is found not to be dislocated but instead merely clicks when the hip is tested this will be followed up and investigations such as scans may be needed. Babies may have to wear a special splint for a while; most cope with these without much problem. Only very few will need an operation.

Congenital dislocation of the hip is more common in girls and in babies born in the breech position.

Conjunctivitis

Conjunctivitis can be caused by infection or allergy such as **hay fever**. Infective conjunctivitis is characterised by a discharge which causes a sticky eye. In allergies the eye tends to be watery.

In both cases the eye is itchy, causing the child to scratch, and the eye may be swollen. In the case of allergy the eye may swell so much that it appears closed.

Conjunctivitis – what you can do

❑ Bathe the eye with warm salty water.
❑ If the eye remains sticky see the doctor.
❑ Infective conjunctivitis is very infectious so the child should have her own towel and nurseries often advise keeping the child at home until the infection is cleared.
❑ Allergic conjunctivitis is treated by anti-histamines. Antihistamine drops are available but tablets or medicine are more effective.

Constipation

Most people will suffer from constipation at some time in their lives and children are no exception. Few people in developed countries eat enough roughage to keep their bowels emptying regularly throughout their lives. As well as roughage we need plenty of fluid to allow the fibre to swell and stimulate the bowel to empty. The normal pattern varies from 2–3 times per day to once every two days. The pattern for breastfed babies can differ from those who are bottle-fed. Breastfed babies may dirty every nappy or may open their bowels very infrequently. They are less likely to develop constipation than babies fed on formula milk.

Some children take longer than others to gain control of their bowels. Some don't like to use a potty and would prefer to dirty their nappy. This is quite normal. Try putting a nappy over the potty, so they sit on the soft nappy, but gradually get used to the idea of sitting on the potty.

You need to be patient about training and not show the child that you are anxious or annoyed. In extreme cases a child may deliberately try not to open their bowels for several days. If this happens the lower bowel becomes filled up with hard faeces and fluid from higher up in the bowel trickles down and causes the child's pants to be dirty. The child will say that he did not know that it happened because he has felt nothing. This is quite different from encopresis, which means that the child empties his bowels in his pants or in inappropriate places. This is much less common than soiling and may be a sign of emotional upset.

Constipation may also happen if the child finds it painful to open his bowels. Haemorrhoids (piles) are very rare in children but anal fissure is fairly common and very painful.

Constipation – what you can do

❏ Give your child more fibre. Oranges are excellent and you can also try other fruits, vegetables, peas and beans. Buy bread with fibre in and remember that many brown breads have no more fibre than white.

❏ Bran is not recommended for very young children, who should be given extra fruit and vegetables plus plenty of water to drink. This is important. Drinking insufficient water is a common cause of constipation.

❏ If a child does not like to drink water dilute squash or fruit juice is fine, but don't overdo fizzy drinks as excessive amounts can cause tummy pain.

❏ If this doesn't work make an appointment at the surgery.

Convulsions

The term 'convulsion' means seizure or fit. A fit is caused by an abnormality of the electrical impulses in the brain. It may start with the person staring into space or with small repetitive movements. The child may fall on to the ground and the movements may become more jerky. She may be quite stiff and may salivate. There may be moaning noises and a change in the colour of the skin to a dusky blue colour. When the jerking stops the child will be drowsy for a while and may seem confused.

In epilepsy fits occur repeatedly and with varying frequency. Epilepsy is sometimes diagnosed using a machine called an electroencephalogram which measures electrical activity in the brain, but more commonly is diagnosed through observation. There are now a great many drugs used to treat epilepsy. In many cases fits stop all together when the child is on treatment. You will come to recognise what is a 'normal' fit and what needs medical attention. Epilepsy can run in some families.

Fits are very frightening to an onlooker who has not seen a fit before. It is important to remain calm and not to panic. Most fits will end within a minute but that minute will seem endless if you are in a panic so do take note of the time.

Fits – what to do

❏ If the child is known to be epileptic move her away from any potentially dangerous object. An epileptic in the middle of a fit would not be able to move away from a fire, for example.

❏ Do not hold the tongue or put anything into the mouth.

❏ When the jerking stops move her into the recovery position (see page 44).

❏ If the child continues to fit for more than a minute call the doctor. Also call the doctor if the fit stops but starts again soon after.

❏ If the child has never had a fit before, call the doctor.

Febrile convulsions

Fits may occur when a child's temperature is very high. The fit may have the features described above. Children over the age of five are less likely to be affected and the risk reduces with age. Sometimes the fit may be the first indication that a child is ill. To prevent a fit it is crucial that efforts to keep the temperature down continue until the fever 'breaks'. This may not happen until 2–3 days after an illness has started. Follow the instructions in the section on fever (page 2) and try to get help for part of the day at least. Nursing a sick child is exhausting.

Always call the doctor for advice. If your doctor is

unable to find a cause for the fever they may advise that admission to hospital would be best.

During the fit follow the instructions given for convulsions (see box opposite). Make sure that you have given the correct amount of paracetamol and keep the child cool. Tepid sponge until the temperature comes down.

Cough

Many children will develop a cough after a cold. This may be a dry cough or a cough which causes phlegm or sputum to be coughed up. The lungs are very good at clearing themselves and most healthy children will get over a cough in about a week. Most coughs are caused by viruses and antibiotics don't help.

Your pharmacist can advise on cough remedies for night time to allow the child to get some sleep. Avoid expectorants at night because they encourage coughing.

Parents should not smoke. Passive smoking can cause a chronic cough in childhood.

Very young children and babies are not good at clearing their throats and parents are often concerned at the rattling noise heard at the back of the throat. The rattle is sometimes transmitted through the lungs and can be felt on the chest wall when you hold the child. By all means take your child to the surgery so that the doctor can listen to the child's chest to check for chest infection but very often the rattle will be found to be due to mucus in the throat which eventually will be coughed up.

Coughs – contact the doctor right away for advice if:

❏ the child is also very breathless
❏ the child appears generally very unwell, e.g. with a very high temperature or severe shivering
❏ the cough started after the child choked on food, e.g. a peanut.

Make an appointment at the surgery if:

❏ the cough lasts more than a week and does not seem to be improving
❏ the cough is worse at night or comes on after exercise; this can be a sign of asthma.

Cradle cap

Cradle cap is a condition which affects the scalp of babies and which causes flaking and a build-up of yellowish crusts on the scalp. It does not upset the baby but parents are understandably concerned about it because it is unsightly.

Cradle cap – what you can do

❏ In mild cases use baby shampoo.
❏ If this doesn't work try applying olive oil at night and washing it off in the morning. This will help in almost all cases but it does need to be continued for some time to keep the scalp clear.
❏ Ask your health visitor for advice.

Croup

Croup is a viral illness which results in a child having difficulty breathing in. Doctors can often make the diagnosis over the phone as there is a very characteristic noise, a little like a sea lion barking. Croup tends to affect young children (i.e. five or under). Older children and adults affected by the same virus might have a sore throat and become hoarse or even lose their voice. This is what is called laryngitis. Even in cases where the voice disappears completely, antibiotics usually do not help. It is helpful to rest the voice but try telling that to a child!

Croup – what you can do

❏ Give paracetamol for any associated fever.

❏ Steam sometimes helps. Try switching on a shower, boiling a kettle or, if you have a tumbler dryer in the home, dampening some towels and putting them in the machine. (Do be very careful not to scald the child with steam or boiling water.)

❏ If there is no improvement after 20 minutes call the doctor.

Epiglottitis is a potentially serious condition which has symptoms similar to croup, but also includes swallowing difficulties and often drooling.

Older children are much less at risk of croup, but always take difficulty in breathing seriously and don't hesitate to call your doctor for advice.

Cystic fibrosis

This is an inherited disease in which a number of body tissues produce an abnormally thick mucus. For example, the lining of the air passages in the lungs normally produces a thin mucus which keeps the lining moist. In cystic fibrosis this is very thick, leading to the air passages becoming blocked and susceptible to infection. The meconium which fills the intestine of the fetus also contains mucus and so a baby with cystic fibrosis may develop a blocked intestine in the first few days of life. The condition also affects the pancreas. This gland produces digestive juices and if it is affected by cystic fibrosis food cannot be digested properly. This means that the child's bowel movements may be loose, fatty and foul-smelling although sometimes constipation will be a problem. The child himself may be undernourished and small for his age.

Cystic fibrosis affects approximately one child in 3,000 in Britain. A test of the amount of salt in the sweat will confirm the diagnosis. There is no cure. However if it is diagnosed early, damage to the lungs can be prevented. Children with cystic fibrosis are very prone to chest infections. These are likely to be bacterial and therefore antibiotics are usually prescribed. Because the mucus in the chest is so thick and sticky the child also benefits from being helped to get it out. Chest physiotherapy involves lying the child head down and patting on the chest with cupped hands to help dislodge the thick phlegm. Parents will usually do this daily to keep the lungs as clear of mucus as possible.

Children affected need special enzyme supplements to help them digest their food and also vitamin supplements because of the poor absorption from the intestine. It also helps if the child eats a diet which is low in fat.

Dandruff

Dandruff is a scaly condition affecting the scalp. The white scales are shed and can be seen in the hair. Sometimes scaly patches are seen on the scalp itself. There may also be itch. In mild cases there is no need to do anything, but in the more severe cases where the scalp is involved coal tar shampoos can be helpful. Cases where there is a large amount of scaling and patches on the scalp may be seborrhoeic **eczema**/dermatitis.

Deafness

In many areas, babies are tested soon after birth. Others have a hearing test at eight months of age. If deafness is suspected the test will often be repeated. If the health visitor is still concerned she will arrange further testing. Parents are very good judges of their children's hearing and audiograms are easy to arrange if there is any suspicion of deafness. Repeated **ear infections** and **glue ear** may lead to hearing loss and subsequent delay in language development so make an appointment at your surgery if you are worried.

Dermatitis

See **eczema**.

Diabetes

Diabetes mellitus is a disease affecting the pancreas. This gland produces the substance insulin, which helps the body use up the sugar which comes from the diet. If there is insufficient insulin glucose builds up in the bloodstream and causes problems for many of the organs of the body.

Insulin-dependent diabetics have to inject themselves with insulin on a regular basis. Insulin cannot be given by mouth. Parents are often concerned at the thought of either giving their child injections or the child giving injections to himself. It is always surprising how even young children cope. If your child is diagnosed with diabetes mellitus it is vitally important that he attends all check-ups and that you learn to keep the strictest possible control over the blood glucose to avoid complications in later life. Uncontrolled blood sugar can affect the circulation, the eyes, the kidneys and other organs in the body. Most young diabetics will use a blood glucose measuring device at home to check the blood glucose level frequently. These are very easy to use even for someone with no medical or nursing training. Children with newly diagnosed diabetes will often be admitted to hospital to be started on insulin.

A 'hypo' refers to an episode of hypoglycaemia or low blood sugar. This may happen if a diabetic has had his normal dose of insulin but for some reason (e.g. a stomach upset) has not had his normal food intake. The child may be sweaty and sleepy or even confused. It is vital that he is given sugar in any form. Special tablets are available which are convenient to carry around. High sugar drinks are also useful for hypos. The one thing that is not appropriate is a sweet which is manufactured for diabetics. These will not raise the blood sugar. An untreated hypo may result in unconsciousness and then it is essential to call a doctor.

The opposite of a hypo is ketoacidosis, which means that the blood sugar is too high. Sometimes diabetes is discovered only when the child develops this condition. There may be drowsiness, abdominal pain and a smell of acetone or vinegar on the breath. Call the doctor right away for advice to distinguish from the following milder cases. In milder cases parents may notice that a child has become excessively thirsty or that the child is visiting the toilet frequently to pass large amounts of urine. In these cases it is easy for your practice nurse to do a stick test in the surgery. This can show it there is sugar in the urine, which would confirm the diagnosis of diabetes.

You may have come across diabetics who use oral tablets. These are usually only suitable for people who have developed diabetes in later life. Children with diabetes will nearly always need insulin to achieve good control over the blood sugar.

Diarrhoea

Diarrhoea means frequent and/or loose bowel motions. It can be due to infections (see **gastro-enteritis**), to intestinal diseases such as colitis (rare in young children) or an inability to digest certain foods.

In cases of digestive problems such as **coeliac disease**

the bowel motions may be fatty, pale and difficult to flush away. They may also be persistently loose and foul smelling, and there may be undigested food in the bowel motion.

A small sample of stool can be sent to the laboratory to test for infection in any case of diarrhoea lasting longer than a few days. Prolonged diarrhoea should always be investigated, and so you should make an appointment at your surgery. If there is blood in the bowel motion contact your doctor right away for advice.

Keep rehydration powders handy (e.g. Dioralyte) to replace the salts lost in diarrhoea. Use correct dosage. It's very important to keep up fluid intake.

Diphtheria

Diphtheria is rarely seen in the UK nowadays, partly because all babies receive immunisation against diphtheria from the age of eight weeks. The illness does not begin acutely and there may not be much of a fever. However it worsens as it progresses. The characteristic feature is a grey membrane in the throat. The fact that it is rare in Britain should not stop parents immunising their children as it is still seen in other countries.

Down's syndrome

This genetic defect is due to a chromosomal abnormality

and affects a child's learning ability. It is diagnosed at birth, if not before.

Dry skin

The skin of babies and children can become dry very easily. This may cause them to scratch because it causes itch, and the skin may appear flaky. In mild cases use baby lotion. If it still seems to disturb the child then it is worth making an appointment at the surgery as the child may be suffering from **eczema**.

Earache

Earache is common after a cold and can be a sign of an ear infection. However, the doctor will often find that the eardrum looks normal and in these cases assume that the pain is due to pressure behind the eardrum caused by a build-up of fluid. Adults and older children will try to 'pop' their ears in the same way as you would in an aeroplane or going up a hill. This will relieve the pressure to a greater or lesser extent. It seems that very young children are not able to do this and this may be why they seem to suffer so much pain when they have an ear infection.

Earache – what you can do

❏ Always give paracetamol at the recommended dose for the age of the child.
❏ Comfort the child. If you have had earache yourself you will know how painful it can be. Children can become very distressed by the pain.
❏ If the pain continues after giving paracetamol, see your doctor at the next available surgery. Antibiotics are sometimes prescribed for ear infections but they do not relieve pain. If there are worrying symptoms other than the earache phone your doctor for advice.

Ear infections

Ear infections often occur after a cold. Most are caused by viruses. The area infected lies behind the ear drum; it is called the middle ear. It connects with the rear nasal passages by way of the Eustachian tubes. The adenoids are tonsil tissue which lie at the bottom of these tubes. If a child seems to contract a lot of ear infections and the hearing becomes affected (see **glue ear**) she may be referred to an ear, nose and throat surgeon who might consider removing the adenoids. Hearing will often be temporarily reduced during an ear infection but will usually go back to normal when the infection has cleared.

Ear infections – what you can do

❏ Follow the directions given for **earache**. Ear infections sometimes need to be treated by antibiotics. However they are not regarded as a medical emergency and an appointment should be made at the surgery. Many parents worry about a perforated eardrum. This can happen with an ear infection and may result in a yellow or green discharge from the ear. Perforated eardrums in children heal up very well and do not usually cause long-term problems with hearing. A perforation may even help the earache because of the release of pressure.

❏ Antibiotics do not prevent perforated eardrum.

❏ Remember that young children frequently develop colds and therefore ear infections, tonsillitis and chest infections are equally common. When deciding on whether or not to remove adenoids (and tonsils) the decision may rest on the number of days lost from school or the extent of deafness.

❏ Adenoid removal does not prevent colds or throat infections.

Ear wax

It is normal to have some wax in the ears. When cleaning children's ears never push a cotton bud into the ear canal as you can actually increase the amount of wax produced. Clean only the outside of the ear.

If you think wax has built up and the child seems to be more deaf than usual, your practice nurse can check for you before treatment. Wax is softened with a drop or two of olive oil twice a day before treatment. Adults and older children can have the wax washed out with a special machine.

Eating problems

Most children will go through phases where they seem to eat very little. It can be quite amazing how little they can eat and still maintain their body weight!

Most children will also go through fussy periods where they seem to want only a very limited range of foods. Even when a child has eaten a wide range of foods as a baby he may suddenly take a dislike to something. This often happens when children start nursery or school and they see other children refusing food.

Eating problems – what you can do

❑ Don't worry. If you need reassurance ask your health visitor to weigh your child. If the child's body weight is within the accepted band for his age and height there is no need to worry.

❑ We all want our children to eat a balanced diet but the worst thing you can do is engage in warfare at the tea table. All children enjoy finding ways to exert some authority as they go through toddlerhood and if they find that Mummy gets in a tizz when they don't eat their greens then suddenly it is fun to not eat greens. It can be exasperating to spend time preparing a meal only to find that he hasn't taken a mouthful, but you must keep calm!

❑ Eating should be an enjoyable social occasion for the whole family. If possible sit down at the table together in the evenings.

❑ Give the reluctant eater small portions and allow plenty of time for him to try the food. Don't cajole, and if he remains reluctant clear the table.

❑ Don't throw the food out unless it is going to be inedible later. Don't give in to requests for snacks, offer the food that has been kept.

It all sounds so simple but it is incredibly difficult to put in to practice. Everyone who cares for your child has to be consistent or your plan will be doomed to failure. And the bad news is that if you win the battle of the tea table you may not win them all! Your toddler is going to try to find an alternative way to exert authority over you. It might be trouble at bedtime or causing you great embarrassment in the supermarket checkout queue.

Obesity is becoming an ever greater problem for our children. Children seem to do less exercise than they used to. Many children do not walk to school any longer because of fears for their safety or simply because the child lives too far from the school. In addition for a variety of reasons many schools find it difficult or impossible to provide after-school sport. Children tend to watch more television and play more computer games than they used to. There is also good evidence that children who are overweight will grow into overweight adults and will be at increased risk of heart disease, diabetes and joint problems. There is also evidence that babies who are fed on milk alone until 15 weeks are less likely to be overweight.

Dealing with a child who is overweight presents a challenge. It is important not to make the child feel guilty or embarrassed about his weight, but at the same time try to encourage healthy eating habits. Many children will choose sweets and crisps rather than fruit but you can with a bit of patience and persistence turn these things into a treat to be enjoyed now and again instead of every day. The whole family may benefit from dietary changes which decrease the intake of fat and increase the amount of fruit and vegetables eaten. Ask your practice nurse if she has some leaflets on healthy eating and if you are still unsure you can have a referral to a dietician. There are lots of books available from your library which will show you that healthy eating need not be expensive.

Eczemas

Eczema and dermatitis mean the same thing – inflamed skin. The tendency for the skin to become dry and inflamed may be inherited and other family members may also have asthma or hay fever. Eczema is a very itchy condition, and children affected will often scratch until their skin appears very red and raw. Eczema often starts in the first or second year of life. It is less common in breastfed babies. One type of eczema can also arise from contact with an irritant, e.g. bleach or washing powders.

Eczema typically affects the skin on the inside of the elbow and behind the knees but any skin area can be affected. Contact eczemas affect the area of contact! Therefore allergy to nickel will affect the area of skin in contact with jewellery and allergy to detergents will often affect the hands. Very mild cases of eczema will simply appear as dry, rough areas of skin with or without itch.

Eczema – what you can do

❏ Avoid obvious irritants in contact eczema.

❏ Use plenty of moisturiser – not the perfumed variety. These are available on prescription for eczema sufferers. Moisturising the skin is the crucial element in eczema treatment. In severe cases it may have to be done several times a day.

❏ Make an appointment at the surgery if moisturisers fail to stop the skin drying out and it becomes red and sore.

❏ In cases of eczema where moisturisers have failed to keep the skin clear doctors often prescribe steroid creams. As steroids can have side effects your doctor will always start with the weakest preparation and only use stronger creams if weak ones don't work. The golden rules with steroids are (1) use as little as you can get away with and (2) when the skin seems to have improved stop or reduce the amount of steroid.

Eczema is a recurring condition! You may not be able to stop it coming back but if you are liberal in your use of moisturisers each time it flares up you may reduce the severity of the attack and possibly also the need for steroids.

All sorts of things can cause flare-ups, from exposure to certain foods and animals to stress.

Many parents ask about homoeopathic remedies for eczema. This is a condition which may respond well to homoeopathic remedies and in many areas of the country this is available free on the NHS.

Enuresis

See **bedwetting**.

Epilepsy

See **convulsions**.

Eye infection

See **conjunctivitis**.

Eyesight

Serious visual problems are usually picked up in the early weeks. The visual system is flexible in the first years, so the sooner treatable problems are found the better. Have all the vision checks you are offered and consult your GP or an ophthalmologist if you are at all concerned.

See **squint**.

Febrile convulsions.

See **convulsions**.

Fifth disease

See **childhood fevers**.

Fits

See **convulsions**.

Flat feet

Children naturally tend to have flat feet compared to adults, who have an arch in their instep. In children often no arch can be seen at all. However when the child stands on tiptoe you will often see the arch. Flat feet are an orthopaedic condition that used to be treated with such things as insoles and even special shoes. Over the years it became apparent that many of these treatments had little effect on the eventual outcome and therefore they were abandoned. Flat feet only very rarely need to be treated.

Flu

See **influenza**.

Foreskin – phimosis and circumcision

A phimosis means a tight foreskin. The foreskin is normally tight at birth and should not be pulled back.

Usually by the time the child is three the foreskin can be gently pulled back. If you feel that it is too tight after this, then make an appointment at the surgery to have it checked by your doctor. In a few cases removal of the foreskin (circumcision) may be needed.

Balanitis is an infection under the foreskin and may be treated by antibiotics. Balanitis causes inflammation, sometimes with a discharge of pus. A child with balanitis may complain of pain when passing urine.

Galactosaemia

See **metabolic disorders**.

Gastro-enteritis

This is an infection of the digestive system which often starts with vomiting and leads to diarrhoea. The exact course of the illness varies depending on the particular 'bug' causing it. Most communities will have minor 'epidemics' of vomiting and diarrhoea from time to time. You may hear of children being off nursery or school with a 'tummy bug'.

Food poisoning is also a form of gastro-enteritis. If diarrhoea occurs on return from a holiday abroad it is especially important to try to obtain stool samples. Take extra care on holiday especially with buffet food, food bought from markets and takeaway food. Wash your hands before eating (with baby wipes if necessary). You and your children can be immunised against typhoid, hepatitis A and cholera if you are going to risky areas.

There are other precautions to take on holidays in hot countries. Drink, and clean your teeth in, bottled water and avoid ice cubes. Avoid drinking milk or milkshakes or eating locally made ice cream, unless it comes pre-packed and you know it's made from pasteurised milk. And steer clear of salads or unpeeled fruit salad (which may have been washed in tap water), rice (unless you know it has just been cooked) or shellfish, which may come from contaminated water. Always remember to take sachets of rehydration salts with you when you go on holiday.

How to treat

❑ Give plenty of fluids. The real danger with these infections is dehydration and young babies are most at risk.

❑ In initial stage of diarrhoea, all foods including cow's milk and artificial milk formulas should be stopped. Breast milk should not be stopped – give oral rehydration fluid (see below) then put to breast until satisfied. After 24–28 hours when symptoms subsiding, you can start normal diet gradually. If child also vomiting take small amounts of oral rehydration solution.

❑ Give paracetamol for fever if required.

❑ DO NOT give anti-diarrhoea mixtures to very young children. Many of them contain chemicals similar to morphine, which can have drastic side effects for babies and small children. At this age diarrhoea can drag on for days on end and if it is very prolonged doctors may occasionally prescribe a safe preparation. However in the early stages it is best simply to persevere with fluids. Doctors do not usually prescribe medicine to stop vomiting.

❑ Rehydration powders are very helpful. These are flavoured, usually come in sachets and are made up with cooled, boiled water. They are designed to replace the salts that are lost in vomiting and diarrhoea. However, many children do not like them because of their slightly salty taste. Try letting them drink through a straw. They won't taste so much this way! And do persevere with drinks that you know your child likes. Remember that rehydration powders do not actually stop vomiting or diarrhoea.

❏ Wash your hands frequently. These illnesses are passed on more readily if there is poor hygiene.

Gastro-enteritis – contact your doctor if:

❏ vomiting is persistent and you are worried about dehydration. Signs to look for are:
  – a dry mouth or tongue
  – the baby's soft spot on the top of the head becomes sunken
  – nappies are dry
❏ the child is very listless or floppy
❏ there is projectile vomiting (this means if the vomiting is very forceful).

There have been worries in recent years about a form of gastro-enteritis caused by a bacterium called *E. coli* O157. *E. coli* has many strains and may be responsible for urine infections and gastro-enteritis. This particular strain has caused more severe illness, often with bleeding in the bowel motions. Always contact your doctor right away if any of your family develop this symptom.

German measles

See **childhood fevers**.

Glandular fever

Most cases of glandular fever occur in teenagers and young adults but this illness can affect younger children. It often starts with a sore throat and fever. The lymph nodes become swollen, the most obvious ones being those under the chin and down the side of the neck. The illness is confirmed with a blood test. Although children will usually recover fully from glandular fever, the recovery period can be prolonged and children will often be tired and listless for several weeks.

Glue ear

Glue ear can be caused by enlarged adenoids and is not always the result of infection, but it often is. After an ear infection the middle ear will usually clear itself of infected fluid and will return to being full of air. However, in a few cases fluid will remain. This can prevent the ear from transmitting sound waves and deafness can result. We call this situation glue ear. Antibiotics will not work because there is no longer any infection. If the ear does not clear itself the child may be referred to an ear, nose and throat surgeon who may insert grommets into the ear drum. Grommets are tiny tubes which sit in the ear drum itself and allow air back into the middle ear. As the eardrum continues to grow the grommets may dislodge and you may find that one has fallen out some months later. Hopefully by this time the glue ear will be cured. Sometimes the **adenoids** will be removed at the same time as the grommets are put in. (See also **ear infection**.)

Haemophilia

See **blood disorders**.

Hand, foot and mouth disease

See **childhood fevers**.

Hare lip

See **cleft palate**.

Hay fever

Hay fever is an allergy to pollen which causes watery, itchy eyes and a watery discharge from the nose with sneezing. The allergy may be to tree, grass and flower pollens and the season of allergy extends from March until September, depending on which pollens the sufferer is allergic to. Treatment in children is usually by antihistamine syrups although nasal sprays are sometimes used. Some children respond to homoeopathic treatment. Treatment which involved desensitisation by giving injections of pollen extract in ever-increasing doses in the hope of reducing the immune reaction was stopped some years ago because of rare but serious anaphylactic reactions.

There have also been concerns about reactions between some antihistamines and other drugs, and for this reason it might be better to take a child with suspected hay fever to see your GP rather than buy antihistamines over the counter. Many GPs, once they have made the diagnosis, will allow your child to have antihistamines on repeat prescription, checking at regular intervals that the drug is still working. You should always tell a doctor or pharmacist issuing any other drug if your child is currently on an antihistamine.

Older children will sometimes have eye drops prescribed. Adults may sometimes have an injection of a steroid at the start of the hay fever season. Many GPs have reservations about using steroids in this way because of potential side effects and it is highly unlikely that a child would ever need this treatment.

Headache

Headache is one of the most common symptoms presenting to GPs, along with backache and tiredness. It is linked to many different illnesses. The commonest form in adults is probably the tension headache which everyone gets from time to time. In children headaches are often linked to fever so most colds, sore throats etc. will be accompanied by a headache. Children may also suffer from **migraine**.

A headache which is felt in the face above and below the eyes could be sinusitis. The sinuses are the hollow parts of the skull. Their lining is similar to that in the nose and they should be full of air. As they connect with the nasal passages they may also be affected when we have a cold. They fill with mucus which can then become infected. The symptoms are facial pain, a feeling of the nose being blocked up, a nasal discharge which is green or yellow and a fever. The face may feel heavy and the pain is worse on movement of the head. The tone of the voice may be changed. Sinusitis will eventually clear on its own but antibiotics can speed up the healing process.

You will not mask more serious symptoms with paracetamol so it is always wise to give the child the correct dose for the child's age. If a headache seems severe and does not settle with paracetamol you should telephone your doctor for advice. In the case of a more recurring, milder headache which responds to paracetamol where the child is otherwise well, make an appointment at the surgery.

Headlice

Most children will pick up headlice at some point in their lives. Contrary to popular belief, they are not a sign of poor hygiene. They can be seen crawling on the scalp and through the hair and can be caught in a fine tooth comb.

Headlice – what you can do

- ❏ Look out for the tell-tale sign of scratching. The eggs or nits are often seen in the hair behind the ears. They look a bit like dandruff but are stuck firmly to the hair.

- ❏ Comb regularly with a fine tooth comb which helps to get rid of nits and damages adult lice, which then may die. Regular combing of wet hair (using 'leave-in' hair conditioner and a fine tooth comb) is the most effective way. It is recommended that this is done once a week at least.

- ❏ Most headlice lotions sold by pharmacists contain malathion. Because of recent worries about the safety of malathion many people have turned to preparations of tea tree oil sold in herbalists shops. Only treat hair when you have actually detected lice or nits. Overuse of preparations is one of the reasons that headlice have become resistant to the available chemicals.

Heart murmurs

When a doctor listens to the heart they can hear two sounds, one after the other in succession. These are the normal heart sounds. If there is an extra sound this is usually called a murmur. A murmur is the sound of the blood flowing through the heart. Heart murmurs may be normal at certain stages of development and there is often a murmur when there is a fever due to the blood rushing through the heart. If your doctor is unsure why the murmur is present they will refer your child for a second opinion from a specialist.

Some murmurs are present at birth and can be a sign that the changes in the baby's heart which should take place at birth have not happened in the usual way. This may mean that blood flows through the chambers of the heart in a different way from normal. Some people describe this as 'hole in the heart'. Many of these holes are not as serious as they sound. The hole in question is on the inside of the heart. It may need to be closed surgically.

Heat-stroke

Never allow your children to become over-exposed to the sun. At best they will suffer mild **sunburn**. At worst they will develop heat-stroke and may be more at risk of skin problems in later life. Use sun hats and T-shirts to keep the sun's rays away from their skin and if they want to swim use a high factor sun block and apply it regularly.

The symptoms of heat-stroke are headache, nausea and vomiting and drowsiness. The child may seem slightly confused. She may be dehydrated.

Heat-stroke – what you can do

❑ Give paracetamol for the headache.
❑ Give plenty of drinks.
❑ Let the child lie down for a while.
❑ If you are worried about excessive drowsiness or confusion call your doctor for advice.

Hepatitis

Hepatitis means inflammation of the liver. This can be caused by a large number of things but in children the commonest causes are viruses and drugs. The most worrying of these are hepatitis B and hepatitis C, which can be transmitted to the baby from the mother during pregnancy. The baby may then carry the virus. Not all carriers of the virus will go on to get hepatitis.

When hepatitis does occur the liver fails to function properly. Certain toxins may accumulate in the blood.

The most obvious feature is jaundice, which means that the skin goes yellow. This is potentially very serious. Hepatitis B and C are both prevalent among drug users who inject their drugs.

Hepatitis A is usually much less serious. This is a diarrhoeal illness and can be contracted by eating contaminated food in the same way as we pick up food poisoning. It only rarely leads to serious complications and it is preventable with good hygiene. There is a vaccine for tourists going to areas where it is common.

Hernias

In a hernia a part of the digestive system is lying outside the cavity of the abdomen where it should be. The commonest form is a protrusion of the intestine through the wall of the abdomen at a point where the muscles have a natural weakness. This may be in the groin, in the scrotum or around the navel (umbilical hernia). Hernias often need surgical treatment to prevent them from becoming stuck outside the abdomen (strangulated hernia). Not all hernias need treatment. Most congenital umbilical hernias (those around the navel) will be left to resolve themselves and will only need surgery if they do not.

A hiatus hernia refers to a part of the stomach pushing through the diaphragm muscle up into the chest. It is relatively rare in children but it can be congenital when it is linked to an unusually short gullet.

HIV

HIV stands for human immunodeficiency virus. This virus is passed from person to person through sexual contact and blood contact (e.g. drug addicts sharing needles, from mother to child in the womb).

Some people who have contracted the HIV virus may go on to develop AIDS which stands for acquired immune deficiency syndrome. In this disease the immune system does not work properly and sufferers are prone to all sorts of infection, which can become serious enough to be life threatening. You will be advised not to breastfeed your baby if you are HIV positive.

There is no cure for AIDS, but the disease can now be actively managed.

Hodgkin's disease

Hodgkin's disease is one of a group of conditions called the lymphomas. They do not usually affect young children, unlike **leukaemia**. In these diseases the lymphatic system is affected by **cancer** cells. The lymphatic system is the body's defence against infection and consists of lymph nodes, which are spread all round the body, and the spleen. In lymphoma these glands may enlarge greatly. Hodgkin's disease is a form of cancer and it is treated with chemotherapy. Great progress has been made in treatment and many children will go into prolonged remission of the disease.

Hydrocephalus

Our brain contains small spaces called ventricles which are filled with fluid. These connect with the fluid around the spinal cord and there should be a continuous circulation of fluid round them. If anything blocks this circulation the fluid will increase in quantity, in turn increasing pressure on the brain tissue. This is known as hydrocephalus.

Hydrocephalus may be caused by meningitis, haemorrhage, tumours or spina bifida or it may occur because of a congenital abnormality. The bones of the skull of a new baby are not joined together and the pressure can push them apart, increasing the size of the baby's head. In an older child where the bones have fused together there will be a severe headache and vomiting caused by the increased pressure. Treatment may be in the form of a shunt which drains the fluid away from the brain into the bloodstream. Some of these may have to stay in place for years and may need to be changed as the child grows.

Hydrocoele

A hydrocoele presents itself as a swelling in the scrotum. It is caused by fluid accumulating in the tissues surrounding the testicle. This is usually on one side only and may present in a young baby. Most will be left to settle by themselves but if the fluid does not seem to be disappearing an operation may be needed.

Hyperactivity

All children may display the signs of hyperactivity but for the vast majority episodes will be short lasting and will usually occur when the child is tired, coming down with an illness, excited or worried about something. In the case of true hyperactivity a child will be restless, inattentive and on the go virtually all of the time. These children find it difficult to learn because they tend to have short attention spans. Reading ability is likely to be lower than average for their age. They behave impulsively and may appear to be excessively impatient. Their behaviour can be annoying, not only to their family but also to other children and they may find friendship difficult.

Many people have suggested reasons for the hyperactivity. These have varied from poor parenting skills to food additives. There does seem to be a genetic element that combines with environmental factors. Poor parenting skills may lead to difficulty in treating hyperactivity, as parents need to learn behaviour therapy techniques, but lack of skills are not now thought to cause the problem.

There is no test for hyperactivity so children need to be interviewed and assessed by skilled staff, who will clearly need to exclude other medical and psychological causes of poor concentration.

Some children do not respond well to behaviour therapy but may benefit from stimulant drugs such as methylphenidate.

Hyperactivity is also known as hyperkinetic disorder and in the United States as attention deficit hyperactivity disorder (ADHD or ADD).

Immunisations

The following table shows the current recommendations for immunisation of children. See over for meningitis C.

When immunisation is given	What it guards against	Injection or by mouth
2 months	polio	by mouth
	Hib diphtheria tetanus whooping cough	one injection
3 months	polio	by mouth
	Hib diphtheria tetanus whooping cough	one injection
4 months	polio	by mouth
	Hib diphtheria tetanus whooping cough	one injection
At 12 to 15 months	measles mumps rubella	one injection
3 to 5 years	measles mumps rubella	one injection
	diphtheria tetanus	one injection
	polio	by mouth
10 to 14 years (sometimes shortly after birth)	BCG (against tuberculosis)	skin test, followed by one injection if needed
13 to 18 years	diphtheria tetanus	one injection
	polio	by mouth

Explanation of the Hib vaccine is given below.

A vaccine against meningitis C was introduced in November 1999. This involves three routine doses of the vaccine by injection at two, three and four months, or a catch-up immunisation for everyone up to the age of 18 over the course of the next year.

Immunisations may be postponed if the baby is suffering from an acute illness when the immunisation is due. However snuffles or a cough where the baby does not have a temperature and is otherwise well will not usually delay an immunisation. Your practice nurse will advise you.

Booster doses may not be given if there has been a severe reaction to a previous dose. It is normal for babies to be grumpy and even have a mild fever after an immunisation. It is also normal for there to be some swelling at the injection site. Always make sure you have paracetamol in the house when your baby has been immunised. Give it at the recommended dose for the age of the child and you will find that it will help her to settle.

Children who suffer from diseases which affect their immune system will not usually be given live vaccines such as polio.

Immunisations will not usually be postponed in premature babies. This means they will start at eight weeks after birth, the same as babies born at term.

There is no good evidence that recent reports linking MMR vaccine to autism and inflammatory diseases of the bowel such as Crohn's disease have been proven.

The Hib vaccine is given to prevent meningitis caused by the organism *Haemophilus influenzae*. This organism causes chest and respiratory infections and before the introduction of the vaccine also caused a substantial number of cases of meningitis each year. These have fallen dramatically after the introduction of the vaccine. However, this vaccine does not prevent meningitis C, caused by the organism *Meningococcus* and this unfortunately causes a number of deaths in children each year. Meningococcal vaccine is given to contacts of cases of meningococcal meningitis. A new vaccine effective against meningitis C has been available since late 1999. It is a step forward in the fight against meningitis although we await the introduction of a vaccine against the B strain, which causes a large number of cases in the UK each year.

For advice on travel vaccines make an appointment with your practice nurse well before the date of travel.

Travel agents vary enormously with regard to the reliability of the information they give. If you have booked a holiday to a risky area, immunise your family according to the current recommendations. Don't take chances simply to avoid jabs. Diseases such as typhoid or hepatitis A can be serious in adults, never mind small children. If your children hate injections why not check out current advice before booking the holiday?

From time to time scares involving vaccines are reported in the press. The worry over MMR and autism is just one. Doctors base their advice on the most recent research information available. When a doctor gives advice on a vaccine they have to weigh up the pros of giving the vaccine against the cons of possible side effects. There are worries that if a large number of children are unimmunised we may see epidemics of such things as measles. Many of us have not seen a child with measles and we forget how ill a sufferer can be. Even worse is the fear that such things as polio may appear again. It is very important when making decisions on immunisation to arm yourself with as much information as you can. Your GP should give you an up-to-date unbiased opinion, but if you still have doubts you can talk to a doctor from the community paediatric team. Your health visitor should be able to arrange this. Never assume that if there is controversy about one vaccine it applies to all of them. The polio vaccine, for example, has been available for a very long time and has never been associated with side effects. (Note, though, that if parents are not immune they are advised not to come in contact with the nappy contents of a newly immunised baby.) At the end of the day it is your decision, but make sure that decision is based on good medical evidence.

Impetigo

Impetigo is an infection of the skin, often the face, which is characterised by yellow crusty patches around inflamed areas. It is very infectious. It often requires an antibiotic so if it doesn't clear up in a day or two make an appointment at the surgery.

Avoid passing the infection to others by washing your hands after contact with the affected areas and letting the child have his own towel.

Influenza

Influenza is an illness caused by a virus. The obvious features of influenza (or flu as most people call it) are very high temperatures and muscle aches. The temperature can be so high that the person feels unable to get out of bed. This phase of the illness is usually quite short – just a couple of days or so. This is followed by exhaustion, which can go on for a few days, and there may be complications such as a chest infection or blocked sinuses. Older children may complain of feeling cold one minute and hot the next. The aches are worst in the large muscle groups such as the shoulders, back, hips and thighs. Headaches are also common.

Flu – what you can do

❏ There is no cure for flu. The temperature should be treated with paracetamol according to the age of the child.

❏ If there are any additional symptoms which cause concern contact the doctor for advice.

❏ Children are not usually recommended to have flu vaccine except in special cases.

❏ In a case of straightforward, uncomplicated flu antibiotics are of no use whatsoever. They will only help if the flu is complicated by, for example, sinusitis.

Insect bites

See the section on bites and stings (page 28).

Intoeing

Intoeing often becomes obvious as the child learns to walk. The toes are seen to point inwards, sometimes causing the child to stumble and fall over. However it rights itself as the child grows and no treatment is needed.

Itch

The medical term for itch is *pruritis*. Itchy skin is most likely to be due to dry skin or **eczema**/dermatitis. It may also be caused by an allergic reaction to something which has been eaten or something which has come into contact with the skin such as washing powder. Infestations such as **scabies** will also cause itch.

Itchy feet may be caused by any skin disease which affects other parts of the body. Itch around the toes could be **athlete's foot** or chilblains. Chilblains are red, tender itchy lumps. Help to prevent your child from contracting these by making sure that she wears warm socks in the winter. Fluctuations in temperature seem to make them worse (e.g. walking on icy pavements followed by blasting the feet with hot air in the car). There are a few rare skin conditions which mainly affect hands and feet.

If your child has an itchy scalp look for **headlice** or scaly patches. Another possible cause is **dandruff**, which could mean seborrhoeic eczema/dermatitis.

Itch around the back passage is known as *pruritis ani*. This could be threadworms or thrush or simply mean that your child is simply having difficulty cleaning herself after she has opened her bowels and needs supervision.

Joint pains

Joint pains may be acute (short-lived) as in flu and other viral illnesses, or chronic (long-standing) as in arthritis. The pains which occur with a viral illness are described as flitting – they move from muscle to muscle and joint to joint. The child will either be hot and flushed or shivery and cold. These pains usually respond to paracetamol.

Arthritis is rare in children. More common are a range of conditions which affect the growing points of bones. These can be quite painful but are rarely serious and disappear when the bones stop growing. (See **osteochondritis**.) Nevertheless, if a child complains persistently of joint pains you should take him to your doctor.

Contact the doctor right away if a child is suddenly unable to put weight on one leg or does not seem to be using one arm. Pain in a single joint associated with a high temperature is also a concern and you should contact your doctor for advice.

There is a form of rheumatoid arthritis which affects children. This is called Still's disease. Rheumatoid arthritis is more likely to affect the small joints of the body such as the hand and wrist than the large joints. This condition needs specialist help in order to try to prevent long-term damage to the joints.

Jaundice

Jaundice means that the skin has a yellow tinge to it; the whites of the eyes are also yellow. This is due to an excess of a pigment called bilirubin, which is measured if a new-born is particularly jaundiced. A degree of jaundice is to be expected in the first few days and may be more severe if a baby is premature. Treatment is by light therapy (phototherapy).

Jaundice occurring in a child at any age should be reported to a doctor straight away. Blood tests will be needed and so the child is likely to be admitted to hospital.

Kawasaki disease

Kawasaki disease is a very rare but potentially very serious disease. It is difficult to diagnose because the features can be very similar to other diseases. It mainly affects children under the age of five.

Kawasaki disease – main features

❏ A very high temperature, more than 40°C, lasting for more than five days.
❏ Inflamed eyes.
❏ Red lips and tongue.
❏ A red rash on the trunk.
❏ Swollen glands. Sometimes this may apply to just one or two glands in the neck.
❏ Later peeling of the skin of fingers and toes.

The above features might not all show at the same time. The underlying problem is an inflammation of small blood vessels. This may lead to one of the serious complications, which is a weakening of the parts of the blood vessels which feed the heart muscle. These weak spots may balloon out and this is what we call an aneurysm. This risk of this complication is greatly reduced if the diagnosis is made and treatment started within ten days of the start of the illness.

Kidney infections

Kidney infections and bladder infections (cystitis) are caused by bacteria getting into the tube which empties the bladder (the urethra) and travelling upwards into the bladder and kidneys. These bacteria are usually ones which live in the skin around the groin area and most come from the bowel. However urine infections are not a sign of poor hygiene and are not infectious. In cases of repeated infection the doctor will recommend tests which are done at a hospital. The simplest of these is an ultra-sound test. This looks for damage to the kidneys or the ureters, which are the tubes that carry the urine from the kidney down into the bladder.

Kidney infections – what to do

❑ There may be a fever. The child may complain of pain or stinging when passing urine. Cloudy or bloodstained urine indicates infection.

❑ If your child seems to be passing urine much more frequently than before or suddenly is wetting the bed or getting up to the toilet in the middle of the night, think of infection.

❑ The kidneys lie just under the rib cage behind the intestines and so an older child with a urine infection may complain of pain in this area of the back.

❑ If you suspect that your child may have a kidney infection or cystitis you should contact your surgery that day. There is a risk that untreated infection may spread up into the kidneys and result in damage.

❑ Give the child plenty of fluids.

A very small child who develops an unexplained fever (i.e. with no cold symptoms such as runny nose or sore throat) may be suffering from a urine infection. Collect a urine bottle from the surgery for children who are old enough to pass urine into a container. For children in nappies you can patiently try to get a 'clean catch' when the child passes urine or you can try using an adhesive bag available from the surgery. You do need to be patient. Remember that it is important to get a sample if at all possible. Not only will the laboratory be able to confirm the diagnosis but the staff will also test the bacteria with antibiotics and provide your doctor with a list of those which have killed the bacteria in the laboratory.

Knock-knees

Knock-knees mean that when the child stands with her knees together there is a gap between the feet. Whether or not treatment is required depends entirely on the size of the gap. Parents are often surprised that treatment is not given for what appear to be marked knock-knees. However, this is a condition which will often right itself and opinion among orthopaedic surgeons is consistent about the degree of deformity which requires treatment.

The same can be said of the opposite condition: bow legs. This means that if a child stands with her ankles together there is a gap between the knees. This used to be seen often as a result of rickets, the condition that resulted from a deficiency of calcium or vitamin D. Nowadays it's rare.

Laryngitis

Laryngitis is an inflammation of the larynx or voice box and causes either hoarseness or croup in young children. It often follows a cold and is usually caused by viruses so antibiotics are rarely of any help. In an adult or older child doctors will usually advise resting the voice but try telling that to a toddler! In the absence of **croup**, laryngitis will usually get better gradually by itself and in a child who is otherwise well there is no need to do anything about hoarseness which lasts a few days. If it goes on for longer than this make an appointment at the surgery.

Leukaemia

See **blood disorders**.

Limp

A limp occurs when there is pain in the foot, leg, hip or back and will usually arise as a result of an injury. If a fracture is suspected then the child must go to A&E. Lesser injuries may cause sprains and strains (see the section on page 47). Young children do not fake limps, at least not for very long. Therefore any limp which arises without injury should be investigated and the child taken to surgery.

Measles

See **childhood fevers**.

Meningitis

This is the one that worries all parents and doctors alike. Cases are still missed because the symptoms can vary from case to case. The organisms are passed from person to person by droplet spread (i.e. in the same way as a cold is spread). The incubation period is 2–3 days. There is usually a fever, the child is often off-colour and there may be vomiting. There may be a rash early on which doctors would call non-specific (i.e. it doesn't have obvious signs of any particular rash and the spots go pale – blanch – on pressure). Later on the rash of meningitis is quite unmistakable. The spots may be pink or purple but the obvious feature is that they do not blanch. You can try this yourself. If you take a glass tumbler and press the side down on many skin blemishes you will see them go pale. If you try it on a mole there is no change in its colour. Meningitis spots are like this. If you ever see a rash like this on an adult or a child you must get medical help immediately. If there is any delay in contacting a GP you should take your child to an A&E unit, preferably in a hospital with a children's ward.

Don't wait for a rash to appear – it may be the last symptom.

Other signs are a stiff neck or back, unusual drowsiness or a change in the sound of a baby's cry. Older children may complain of pain when they look at a light (photophobia). The child may be very irritable.

One of the problems with meningitis is that the early signs are the same as those of a fever. On an average night on call a GP may see several children with fevers. Although your doctor will think about meningitis and probably test for it, a child who is in the early stages may not show the signs until some hours later.

Don't be afraid to ask your doctor about the signs to look for and if your child's condition seems to be deteriorating call back. Thankfully meningitis is extremely rare. If we all remain vigilant we can help make it rarer still.

Meningitis checklist

❏ severe headache
❏ high temperature
❏ stiff neck
❏ vomiting
❏ drowsiness
❏ sensitivity to light
❏ rash as described as above.

Metabolic disorders

There are an enormous numbers of disorders of metabolism. In many of these conditions a chemical process in the body malfunctions or fails to function. This could be due to a lack of a particular chemical. Most of these conditions are determined by genes. This means that the condition is present from birth and so the group of conditions is also known as 'inborn errors of metabolism'.

Phenylketonuria is one such disorder. A test for this forms part of the Guthrie test done on all newborn babies by midwives. In this condition there is a deficiency of an enzyme, which leads to a build up of one of the protein 'building blocks' called phenylalanine in the bloodstream. This leads to mental subnormality and growth retardation. The condition, once detected, can be helped by restricting phenylalanine in the diet, using a special diet designed for the children.

In galactosaemia a deficiency of an enzyme leads to an accumulation of galactose in the blood. Babies become ill as soon as they start drinking milk. Treatment is by the exclusion of milk from the diet.

Migraine

A migraine is a headache which occurs in episodes. It can be quite severe and the sufferer may have to lie down in a darkened room until it passes off. Some children may be able to pick up warnings that a migraine is about to happen. These include visual changes such as wavy lines in their visual field, sparkles or blurring of their vision. There may be a time delay between the warning sign and the headache. Some children will vomit or feel nauseated. Migraine headaches may run in families.

Migraine – what you can do

❏ Even if you have migraines yourself and are convinced that your child is also a sufferer, you should still see your doctor to confirm the diagnosis. By all means give your child paracetamol if he complains of a headache.

❏ If the headache does not settle with paracetamol, telephone your doctor for advice.

❏ Migraines may well respond to simple painkillers and many migraine sufferers will find that if the painkiller is taken soon after the onset of symptoms that is all they will need.

❏ There are other more specific treatments available on prescription and some of these are suitable for children. If you have migraine treatment on prescription from your doctor never assume that it will be OK for your child to take it.

❏ Some find that certain foods or activities trigger a migraine. Cheese and chocolate are well-known ones but others may become obvious.

Moles

It is important not to ignore changes in moles and if you are worried about a mole make an appointment at the surgery. This cancer is called malignant melanoma.

Mole changes that are worrying:

- ❏ a change in size
- ❏ the mole becoming raised up from the skin
- ❏ a change in the colour of a mole
- ❏ new moles appearing round the circumference of an existing mole
- ❏ bleeding from a mole.

Malignant melanoma is rare in children. However, with increased exposure to the sun during foreign holidays the number of cases in adults is going up and this may apply to children in future years. See **heat–stroke** for advice.

There is evidence that episodes of sunburn in childhood can increase the risk of skin cancer in adulthood. It is vital that children are protected from the sun. Keep children covered when they are not swimming and use sun block, reapplying it often. Families who ski should remember that snow reflects the sun's rays and exaggerates its effects. Look for small tubes of sun block and lip sun block which a child can take with them to a holiday club or ski lesson.

Molluscum contagiosum

This is a crop of small, shiny, raised spots, often appearing as a small group on one part of the body. It is mildly infectious and is passed through close contact. It is treated for cosmetic reasons if the spots are on a conspicuous area, but treatment is not necessary if the crop is small and the spots are not bothering the child. They will go by themselves eventually.

Mumps

See **childhood fevers**.

Muscular dystrophy

This refers to a group of conditions which are usually inherited and which affect children. The muscles do not work properly and children may have difficulty walking and climbing stairs. Duchenne muscular dystrophy is a sex-linked condition and the gene is recessive; it affects boys but girls can be carriers.

The disease is progressive, which means that the muscle malfunction gets worse as the child gets older. Many children affected will not grow to adulthood.

Nappy rash

This is caused by the skin of the nappy area coming into contact with urine or faeces and may be complicated by **thrush** in some cases.

Nappy rash – what you can do

❑ Try to leave the nappy off. Small babies love to kick and stretch their legs when their nappies are taken off and will happily lie on a changing mat for a little while. It may be more difficult with someone who is on the move, at least in winter, when she can't run around outside.

❑ Change nappies often. It doesn't matter whether you use terries or disposables, the same rule applies. Apply small amounts of barrier cream. Large quantities can affect the absorption of disposable nappies. Be extra cautious at any time when your baby's diet is changing or if your child develops diarrhoea or loose bowel movements.

❑ Use baby lotion, lotion wipes or gentle baby soap to clean the skin.

❑ If all this has failed ask your doctor to prescribe an anti-fungal cream to apply to the skin.

Pertussis

See 'whooping cough' under **childhood fevers**.

Pneumonia

See **chest infections**.

Polio

Polio, short for poliomyelitis, is an illness caused by a virus which is passed on via the digestive system. The virus multiplies in the nervous system and the symptoms may range from virtually nothing at all to full-blown paralysis. Polio is still a big problem in some developing countries and travellers should always make sure they are immunised. It is rarely seen in the UK now but if immunisation levels were to drop it could begin to cause problems again.

Prickly heat

This occurs during hot weather and is made worse by exposure to the sun. It is extremely itchy and there may be redness of the skin.

You can treat it with antihistamines or hydrocortisone cream 1%, available from your pharmacist. Always remember the golden rules with hydrocortisone or other steroid creams: use very sparingly, don't apply it to the face unless advised to do so by your doctor and stop using it as soon as the condition gets better.

Pyloric stenosis

The pylorus is the exit from the stomach into the first part of the intestines, the duodenum. 'Stenosis' is the medical term for a narrowing, so pyloric stenosis means that the outflow from the stomach is partially blocked. This may cause projectile vomiting – vomiting that is so forceful that it travels a distance and may even hit the opposite wall of the room! Babies with pyloric stenosis may need to have a small operation to relieve the blockage.

Ringworm

Ringworm is a fungal infection which causes infections on the skin. It has a rather unfortunate name conjuring up an image for some people of worms. There are no worms in ringworm. It is no worse than having athlete's foot. The main difference is that athlete's foot affects sweaty areas and ringworm usually affects dry skin areas. The patches are often in a ring and grow outwards. They may be itchy.

Pets can suffer from this and are sometimes the source of the infection. It is an infectious condition that responds to treatment, albeit slowly. You can buy the cream used for it, clotrimazole, over the counter and your pharmacist can advise you about treatment.

The medical name for fungal skin infections is tinea. There is a similar infection called *Tinea versicolor* which causes small scaly patches, again on dry skin. This also responds to anti-fungal creams but has the unfortunate effect of affecting the skin's ability to tan. Affected areas stay pale, but will go back to normal some months after treatment.

Rubella

See **childhood fevers**.

Scabies

Scabies is caused by a tiny mite which burrows into the skin. It is very infectious and causes intense itch. It tends to be worse in areas where the mite is trapped, such as waistbands and between the fingers. It is sometimes treated by a cream or lotion which is available on prescription so you can make an appointment at the surgery. However treatment is also available without prescription; if you can't make it to the surgery ask your pharmacist for advice.

Scalds

See the section on burns (page 32).

Scarlet fever

See **childhood fevers**.

Shingles

Shingles is rare in children. It is caused by the **chickenpox** virus and you can't have shingles until you have had chickenpox. The virus affects one skin nerve; it appears on one side of the body only and causes a crop of blisters very similar to chickenpox but in a cluster. It can be very painful, and if present on the face can cause eye damage, so if you do see a crop of blisters on your child's skin, see your doctor that day.

Sickle cell disease

Sickle cell disease is an inherited condition found in people of West African or Afro-Caribbean descent.

The substance which transports oxygen around the

body is called haemoglobin. People with sickle cell disease have a different type of haemoglobin, which takes on a different shape when it gives up its oxygen to the tissues. The red cells containing the haemoglobin become sickle shaped. This results in their being broken down more quickly than normal by the organ called the spleen, which means that sufferers frequently become anaemic. Also the abnormally shaped cells can cause blockages of blood vessels which lead to episodes of pain in the limbs or abdomen. Episodes may last a few days and should be treated with painkillers such as paracetamol.

Slapped cheek disease (Fifth disease)

See **childhood fevers**.

Sore throats

Sore throats can be caused by inflammation of the tonsils (tonsillitis), the pharynx (pharyngitis) or the larynx (laryngitis). The tonsils are the spongy-looking areas on either side of the arch as you look at the back of the throat and the pharynx is the bit beyond the arch – the back of the throat. You can't see the larynx because it is too far down, but you know you have laryngitis if you are hoarse. Younger children may develop **croup** if their larynx is affected.

All sore throats may be accompanied by a fever, nasal congestion and a cough. There will also be **swollen glands**. Tonsillitis will generally be the worst of the three, causing a child to be generally unwell.

Sore throats – what you can do

❏ First of all, treat as for a fever (see page 2). If the child is otherwise fine he may not need to see a doctor at all and you will be able to treat the sore throat yourself.

❏ The vast majority of sore throats are caused by viruses and antibiotics make absolutely no difference to the progress of the disease. Doctors may decide to use antibiotics to treat a true tonsillitis (i.e. where the tonsils are very enlarged with white discharge) but pharyngitis does not respond to antibiotics and it only lasts a few days.

❏ In older children painkilling lozenges may help. Your pharmacist can advise on suitable ones to buy over the counter.

❏ All sore throats cause pain on swallowing. If your child has difficulty in swallowing contact your doctor.

Speech problems

If your baby seems to be slow in talking, ask your health visitor to book a hearing test. This is especially worth doing if your child has had a lot of ear infections, which can lead to temporary loss of hearing.

Some children have difficulty pronouncing certain sounds because the mouth and organs of speech aren't fully mature until a child is six year old. If you are worried that difficulty in pronouncing words is making it difficult for your child to communicate effectively, ask your doctor or health visitor to refer you to a speech therapist for an assessment.

Spina bifida

This is a disorder of the spinal cord. When the spinal cord, sometimes known as the neural tube, forms in the fetus it may be malformed. This can happen at any level from the brain stem down. With spina bifida aperta, part or all of the spinal cord may remain open and nerves below this level will not function. The baby is born with a raw swelling over the spine. The end results can be partial or complete paralysis of the legs, loss of sensation below the level of the spina bifida and problems with bladder function. There may also be **hydrocephalus**. Lesions will be closed surgically in a specialist unit if possible.

All pregnant women and women planning a pregnancy have been encouraged to take supplements of folic acid in the prenatal period and in the early months of pregnancy as this reduces the risk of giving birth to a baby with spina bifida.

Squint

During the first six months of life, a baby's eyes don't always follow each other. After that time they start to move together. Most infant squints appear between the ages of two and four. A child's eye may squint inwards (convergent squint) or outwards (divergent squint). A squint would usually cause double vision, but the brain copes with this by suppressing the image from one eye. This can become permanent, so it is important to seek advice for squints at any age, other than very brief episodes. Your doctor, child health clinic or optician can refer your child to an orthoptist who is a specialist in squints.

Still's disease

See **joint pains**.

Sunburn

Take great care not to let your child's skin redden in the sun, but if it does happen treat sunburn with calamine lotion and cool baths. Paracetamol is also helpful for pain. Consult your doctor if the skin has blistered. See also **heat-stroke**.

How to prevent sunburn

❑ Keep the child out of the sun.
❑ All babies and young children should be kept out of the sun during the middle of the day.
❑ Use hats and long-sleeved clothes to protect the skin and high factor suncreams.

Swollen glands

The glands which most people refer to when they describe swollen glands are those under the chin. These glands are known to doctors as lymph nodes and they are part of the body's defence against infection. There are lymph nodes all over the body, some just under the skin and some deep inside the body. As soon as an infection is contracted the local glands start to work. In some viral infections glands all over the body will swell.

Swollen glands on their own do not constitute a diagnosis and your doctor would try to identify the cause of them. In most cases this will be a virus which requires no treatment other than that for fever (see page 2). The glands will usually reduce to the size of a baked bean after a week or two. Glands which remain enlarged for longer than this should be checked by a doctor.

Talipes

See **club foot**.

Teething

The age at which babies acquire their first teeth varies enormously. A few are born with teeth while others may not have any teeth until they are over a year old. The degree to which a baby suffers as the teeth erupt also varies a great deal. Some may be perfectly OK while others can be very grumpy. Teething is blamed for many other symptoms but most of these cannot really be attributed to the teeth (e.g. the drooling associated with teething may produce a rash around the chin and neck but not elsewhere). Teething does not give rise to diarrhoea.

Teething – what you can do

❏ Apply painkilling gels to the gums. These are available from your pharmacist.
❏ Give paracetamol appropriate to the baby's age.
❏ Accept help from relatives who offer it. If your baby is upset by teething, it can be a fraught time.

Temperature

See the section on fever (page 2).

Threadworms

Threadworms, like headlice, are a common problem of childhood and are not a sign of poor hygiene. The worms are white and about half an inch long and live in the bowels. They come out of the back passage at night to lay their eggs on the skin, causing the child to have an itchy bottom. The child scratches and eggs get stuck under the nails where they stay until the child passes them on to someone else the next day – pretty disgusting really but easily treated!

Threadworms – what you can do

❏ Anyone over the age of two can take a dose of piperazine 100mg available from your pharmacist or on prescription. It is sensible to treat the whole family and to repeat the dose after ten days if worms are still seen in the bowel motions.

❏ Teach your child to wash her hands often.

❏ Keeping fingernails short and wearing cotton underpants at night helps.

Thrush

The organism which causes thrush is *Candida albicans*, a yeast. Thrush affects mainly the mouth, the vagina and the groin area. See **nappy rash**.

Oral thrush appears as small white spots on the baby's tongue and the inside of the lips and cheeks. If these are wiped off there is a raw red area underneath. Thrush causes the mouth to be tender and will make feeding from a teat difficult.

If your baby suffers from recurrent oral thrush and you are using feeding bottles and teats, try another method of sterilisation other than tablets or sterilising fluid (e.g. steam sterilising). Some cases of thrush can be caused by an imbalance of the body's 'normal' bacteria.

The same applies to recurrent vulval thrush in girls. The two commonest causes are antibiotics and bubble bath/bath oils which again upset the balance of bacteria. Vulval thrush appears as a thick white or cream discharge often with intense itching – especially at night.

There are two treatments available on prescription for oral thrush, a suspension with a dropper and an oral gel. For vulval thrush your doctor will prescribe anti-fungal cream for children.

Thyroid gland

The thyroid gland is situated in the neck just under the Adam's apple. It secretes a hormone called thyroxine which regulates the rate at which many of the processes in the body work. If it is overactive the heart rate may go up, and the person may lose weight and be edgy and jumpy. If the gland is underactive the opposite happens. Thyroid disease is rare in children. However it is possible for a baby to be born with no functioning thyroid tissue and this is not likely to be noticed at birth. It can lead to mental retardation so a test for thyroid function forms part of the Guthrie test done on newborn babies by midwives.

An underactive thyroid gland is treated with thyroxine. This is not a drug but a substance chemically identical to the natural hormone.

Ticks

Ticks are sheep parasites. If you live near a sheep farm or if you go on holiday to an area where there are sheep you may be bitten by one of these small insects. You may not feel anything at the time but ticks are blood suckers and gradually their body swells to the size of a grain of sweetcorn. When a tick is removed it is important to remove all of it, including the mouthparts. Shepherds use a lighted cigarette but this method is not recommended for children! The safest way is to smother the tick in Vaseline or apply surgical spirit. The tick should then let go and can be removed with tweezers.

It is not recommended that antibiotics are used routinely for tick bites. Obviously if a bite site begins to look red and inflamed you should make an appointment at the surgery.

Lyme disease is a rare complication of tick bites. It begins with a rash of spots which start as small red swellings and slowly enlarge into red rings with a raised edge. These can last from a few days to a few weeks. The sufferer may also be generally unwell with joint pains. It can progress to more serious complications and should be treated with antibiotics.

Tonsillitis

See **sore throats**.

Toothache

Toothache is often caused by dental caries or tooth decay. To help prevent decay from occurring children should be taught to brush their teeth from an early age. They should be helped until you are certain that they are capable of doing it thoroughly by themselves.

It is also important to check that your child is not using too much toothpaste. Using large amounts of fluoride-containing toothpaste can permanently stain the teeth. A small pea-sized amount of toothpaste is all that's needed for a child.

As well as ensuring that your child is brushing her teeth regularly and effectively you should try to limit the amount of sugar-containing food and drinks in your child's diet. Many fruit squashes and drinks specifically marketed for children have high sugar levels. Don't allow your child to make up her own squash until you are certain that she is able to dilute it correctly.

Toothache – what you can do

❏ Make sure you are registered with a dentist. Dentists are only obliged to offer emergency treatment to patients registered with them.

❏ Always try paracetamol at the recommended dose for the age of the child. This will be sufficient for most mild toothaches.

❏ Contact your dentist if toothache is severe. After surgery hours you will usually get an answering machine giving you instructions on how to contact the dentist. If you are requested to leave a message the dentist will ring you back later. All NHS dentists have to provide an emergency service for their patients.

❏ If you do not have a dentist, telephone your local A&E unit, where there may be an emergency dental service the next day.

❏ Your GP does not have the means to make a diagnosis in dental problems and will only provide pain relief in an absolute emergency when a dentist cannot be contacted. Because they have no training in dental problems, GPs will not usually prescribe antibiotics unless a diagnosis of abscess is very obvious.

Toxocariasis

This infection is caused by an organism called *Toxocara* and is picked up from the faeces of dogs and cats, where the organism's eggs are found.

This disease may cause blindness but it is preventable. All dogs and cats should be wormed regularly; ask your vet for advice. Many people irresponsibly allow their pets to foul public places. If you have a dog make sure that you clean up behind it.

Toxoplasmosis

Toxoplasmosis is an infection caused by an organism called a protozoan. This may be found in raw or undercooked meat and also in the faeces of cats and sometimes dogs. In the vast majority of cases, infection does not produce any symptoms and in the cases where there are symptoms, these may be vague. Swollen glands may occur, mainly in the neck, and sometimes there is fever and sore throat.

If you think you might be at risk of toxoplasmosis you can have a blood test to check. There are antibiotics available for cases contracted in pregnancy – because, if picked up by a pregnant woman, toxoplasmosis can be passed on to the unborn baby and this can have devastating effects such as eye problems leading to visual impairment, epilepsy or mental retardation. Pregnant women should not eat undercooked meat or clean the cat litter tray.

In many cases of toxoplasmosis there are few or no symptoms. This is why it is especially important to try to prevent contraction of the illness in pregnancy by adhering to the advice above. Up to a third of babies born to mothers infected in pregnancy may be infected themselves. Many adults in the UK will already have antibodies because of past infection and in fact will not realise that they have been infected.

In the non-pregnant, recovery occurs without any treatment in the vast majority of cases.

Travel vaccines

The advice varies depending on the country you are visiting and even on whether you are visiting an urban or rural area. Don't depend on your travel agent to advise you. Most travel agents will try to give good advice but they are not provided with current recommendations as frequently as practice nurses are. Practice nurses will give you the latest available advice.

Children hate injections! Many parents book holidays without realising that vaccines are recommended so check with your nurse first.

Remember that you may have to have immunisations a few weeks before your holiday so book an appointment in plenty of time. Malaria tablets also have to be taken in advance of the trip and continued after you have arrived home. Yellow fever immunisation is not available at all surgeries.

Tuberculosis

This has now become a rare disease in developed countries, thanks to good public hygiene, antibiotics and immunisation. It is still very common in developing countries though, and we see occasional cases in Britain. It is more likely in overcrowded living conditions. All children in the UK are offered a test to check if they have been exposed to TB and subsequently an immunisation. This is done around the age of 13–15, depending on the area in which you live, and is usually organised by community paediatric doctors through the school health service.

Undescended testes

The testes or testicles develop inside the body and descend into the scrotum before birth. Baby boys are checked at birth and at eight weeks for undescended testes. If testes do not descend into the scrotum by themselves an operation may be needed to prevent problems in later life.

Urine infection

See **kidney infections**.

Urticaria

Urticaria is an allergic condition which presents as a blotchy rash. The rash can resemble nettle stings. It is often due to food or drinks and may be due to an additive, say in a fizzy drink. GPs often have to rack their brains to come up with the culprit but the treatment is usually straightforward – antihistamines (and avoidance of the culprit, of course!). See the section on rashes on page 9.

Verruca

A verruca is a wart which develops on the sole of the foot and therefore it is usually flat. Most verrucas are not painful and it is not fair to subject a child to painful treatment for a condition which will eventually get better by itself. If the verruca is causing pain, it can be treated either by applying salicylic acid every day (available from the pharmacist) or by freezing with liquid nitrogen or a similar substance at the surgery. It usually needs to be treated several times and the treatment is often painful.

Most verrucae disappear after a year or two. They are only very slightly infectious, and they do not cause any harmful effects anywhere else on the body.

Children should not be prevented from swimming because of a verruca. It is tremendously important for safety that children learn to swim. Just cover the verruca with a waterproof sticking plaster.

Viruses

Viruses are tiny, microscopic organisms which cause infection. There are millions of different types and many different strains of each type. Patients get fed up with doctors telling them 'It's just a virus', but there are so many viruses that most of the illness that GPs see is in fact due to them.

Viral illnesses range from straightforward colds and sore throats to more serious and even life-threatening HIV and hepatitis B. We have very few effective treatments for viral illnesses. Antibiotics do nothing at all unless a patient has developed a secondary bacterial illness on top of their viral illness (e.g. sinusitis after a cold).

The drugs which are effective against viruses are used mainly in hospital for in-patients who have poor resistance to infection because of other illnesses. Anti-viral drugs are never used against colds and flu in otherwise healthy people. We cannot risk viruses becoming resistant to the few anti-viral drugs available, in the way that many bacteria have become resistant to penicillin and other antibiotics.

Viruses can cause fever, headache, muscle aches, sore throat, earache, hoarseness, cough, swollen glands, rashes, tiredness, poor appetite, vomiting, diarrhoea, cold sores, joint pains, chest pains and many other symptoms – which explains why doctors make the diagnosis of a viral illness so often. The good news is that otherwise healthy adults and children have a natural defence against these organisms and the vast majority of viral illnesses will disappear without causing damage to the tissues of the body.

Viruses – what you can do

❑ With viruses you treat the symptoms.
❑ Treat fever as described in the section on fever (page 2).
❑ Treat pain with paracetamol.
❑ Call the doctor if there are any of the worrying signs listed in the section on fever.

Vomiting

Vomiting can be caused by many different illnesses in children. Almost any illness which causes a fever can cause vomiting. However the most common cause of prolonged vomiting which doctors see is **gastro-enteritis**.

In all cases of vomiting the main priority is maintaining a good intake of fluids. Even when vomiting is very persistent it is essential to keep encouraging a child to drink. Any fluid will do, except ones with large amounts of glucose (e.g. high-energy drinks) and drinks which are very acidic such as fruit juices. See page 114 for more information.

The next priority is the fever, which should be treated as advised above. Signs of dehydration in a baby or toddler include a dry mouth or tongue, skin which has lost its elasticity, a sunken soft spot on the top of the head in a child under the age of 18 months and dry nappies. If an older child starts to vomit look for similar signs in the mouth and skin but also take notice of the number of times the child needs to pass urine and how much is passed. Telephone your doctor for advice if more than 12 hours go by without the child passing urine or there are any of the other signs of dehydration above. However, it is unlikely that a child who has vomited once or twice has dehydration. Doctors are unable to prescribe drugs to stop vomiting in young children.

There are a variety of drugs available to treat children who suffer from travel sickness. Ask your pharmacist for advice.

Warts

See **verruca**.

Whooping cough

See **childhood fevers**.

Worms

See **threadworms**.

7

The team that's here to help

What is care in the community?

Health care in the community means care outside hospitals, at a clinic or in your home.

And what is meant by primary & secondary care?

Primary care is your first port of call when you need medical care, whoever that might be.

Secondary care is another term for specialist care. It's who you see when you are referred to experts.

There are many people and organisations 'in the community' that can help you with family health problems.

Family doctor

Your family doctor or 'general practitioner' (GP) is usually the first person you will see when you are ill.

GPs in the UK are contracted by the National Health Service to provide 24-hour care for their patients. Most doctors will work in a group practice so that they can share night emergency cover and therefore don't have to be on duty 24 hours a day seven days a week. Many doctors have taken this further by setting up on call services with all night centres for patients to visit if they need emergency care. Doctors will still visit if a patient is unable, for medical reasons, to attend the all night centre.

UK GPs have on average just under 2,000 patients each to look after. To enable them to do this effectively, most arrange their working day into a morning surgery followed by home visits and paperwork followed by an afternoon or evening surgery. Few surgeries can afford the luxury of having a doctor sitting around waiting for emergencies and so when a doctor does attend an emergency this oftens means the patients with booked appointments may be kept waiting.

This also explains why most surgeries will ask you to request home visits early in the day except in the case of sudden emergencies. Doctors in both cities and rural areas need to plan their visiting route if at all possible to avoid wasting time making the same journey twice.

If you need to speak to your doctor, but don't need an appointment, ask the receptionist when it would be convenient to speak to the doctor. Most doctors will be happy to break off from doing their paperwork to give telephone advice to a patient but might feel unhappy to interrupt another patient's consultation.

If you are on holiday in another part of the UK you can see a GP if you need to without charge. Look in the yellow pages under Doctor for the telephone number of a surgery.

We all hope that we will never need the help of the emergency services but if your child suddenly became ill would an ambulance staff or your doctor be able to find their way easily to your home? Ambulance and fire crews waste precious minutes searching for houses with either no number plates or illegible number plates and people dealing with an emergency in their home are often in too much of a panic to give coherent directions to their home. It has also become fashionable to address a house by its name only but if you live in such a house do the staff of your local ambulance station know where it is? Take a look at your house at night and choose a conspicuous place to position a legible number (or name). It could save you or your child's life.

Dentist

All children in the UK are entitled to free dental treatment. However you should register all of your family with a dentist to ensure continuity of treatment and to make sure that you will receive emergency treatment if you need it. Your dentist is obliged to give 24 hour care for dental problems but is not obliged to treat people who are not on his or her practice list. Don't wait until you have toothache before registering.

Practice nurse

Your practice nurse works closely with your GP to provide primary care services. She will be responsible for providing both childhood immunisations and travel immunisations. She will apply dressings, treat minor injuries and burns and give advice on diet and lifestyle. She may run her own specialised clinics such as an asthma clinic or diabetic clinic. Some nurses have taken extra training to allow them to prescribe and give advice on minor illnesses. These nurses are called nurse practitioners and they work to strict protocols when they prescribe drugs.

Health visitor

Your health visitor will provide advice on all aspects of baby and child care and he or she will be the first person to contact if you have problems with your child's sleeping pattern, eating, toilet training, development and many other issues. If your health visitor feels that referral may be needed she will advise you to see your doctor. A health visitor will visit all newborn babies within the first fortnight of life. She will also be responsible for baby and child clinics where check-ups are done.

Midwife

Your midwife will be responsible for your care during pregnancy and for the care of you and your baby for the first ten days after birth although she may, in some cases, carry on visiting for longer than this if a mother needs longer term care. She will help you to decide how to feed your baby and will deal with any problems immediately after birth. If you decide on a home delivery she will visit you at home and attend you as soon as you contact her to let her know that you are in labour.

Practice receptionist

Receptionists have a difficult job trying to juggle the availability of doctors and nurses with all the demands that are made of them. Sometimes it is necessary for them to ask for medical details and this can cause offence. However if they know that the doctor is already dealing with an urgent case they do have to gather as much information as possible to enable the doctor to decide on the level of priority each case should receive. Receptionists are bound by the same rules of confidentiality as everyone else at the surgery. Don't forget that they file all the letters and type referrals and many of the doctors' clinical records so they do have access to a great deal of confidential information. Any breach of confidentiality would be treated as harshly as if a doctor had committed it and so you can be sure that information given to them is treated in a confidential manner.

8

Useful organisations

National Childbirth Trust
Alexandra House
Oldham Terrace
London W3 6NH
Tel: 020 8992 8637
Fax: 020 8992 5929

Action for Sick Children
300 Kingston Road
Wimbledon Chase
London SW20 8LX
Tel: 020 8542 4848
Fax: 020 8542 2424
Advice and information for parents with children in hospital.

Association for Spina Bifida and Hydrocephalus
ASBAH House
42 Park Road
Peterborough PE1 2UQ
Tel: 01733 555988

British Diabetic Association
10 Queen Anne Street
London W1M 0BD
Careline 020 7636 6112

Cleft Lip and Palate Association
(CLAPA)
235–237 Finchley Road
London NW3 6LS
Tel: 020 7431 0033
Fax: 020 7431 8881

Coeliac Society
PO Box 220
High Wycombe
Buckinghamshire HP11 2HY
Tel: 01494 437278

Contact–a–Family
020 7383 3555
Helping families of children with special needs.

Down's Syndrome Association
155 Mitcham Road
London SW17 9PG
Tel: 020 8682 4001

Health Information Service
Tel: 0800 665544 (England and Wales)
Tel: 0800 224488 (Scotland)
Tel: 0845 7581929 (Northern Ireland)
A national network of NHS-funded helplines providing
free, confidential information on illnesses and treatments,
keeping well, using health services, rights and complaints.
Around 200 lines in 26 centres.

ParentAbility
Disabled Parents Network
PO Box 5876
Towcester
NN12 7ZN

REACH
25 High Street
Wellingborough
Northamptonshire
NN8 4JZ
Tel: 01933 274126
The association for children with hand/arm deficiency.

SCOPE
6 Market Road
London N7 9PW
Tel: 020 7619 7100
Helpline: 0800 626216
Mon–Fri 9am–9pm
Sat–Sun 2–6pm
Fax: 020 7436 2601
Help for children with cerebral palsy and their carers.

Sickle Cell Society
54 Station Road
Harlesden
London NW10 4UA
Tel: 020 8961 7795/020 8961 4006
National charity for Sickle Cell Sufferers.

Twins and Multiple Births Association
(TAMBA)
Harnott House
309 Chester Road
Little Sutton
Ellesmere Port
CH66 1QQ
Tel: 0151 348 0020
Helpline: 01732 868000
Mon–Fri 7pm–11pm; 10am–11pm at weekends

Index

dandruff 98, 133
deafness 98
dehydration, signs of 167–8
delirium 8
dental care
  abscesses 52
  teaching children to brush
    teeth 160
  and toothache 160–1
dentists 161, 172
dermatitis see eczema
diabetes 49, 99–100
dialling 999 13–14, 16
  and breathlessness 74
  and choking babies 34
  and heart massage 46
diarrhoea 51, 100–1, 166
  and gastro-enteritis 113
  mixtures 114
diet
  avoiding constipation 56,
    89, 90
  gluten-free 83, 84
  and metabolic disorders
    141
  and migraine headaches
    142
diphtheria 101
  immunisation 127
doctors see GPs (general
  practitioners)
dog bites 28
dogs, and toxocariasis 162
Down's syndrome 101–2
drowning 38
drugs
  anti-viral 166
  aspirin 6
  giving medicine to your
    child 17–20
  steroids 60, 109, 118, 147
  see also antibiotics;
    antihistamines;
    paracetamol
dry skin 102
Duchenne muscular
  dystrophy 144

E. coli 115
ear drops 20
ear infections 2, 50, 52, 84,
  98, 103–4, 152
ear thermometers 3
ear wax 105
earache 102–3, 104, 166

eating problems 105–8
eczema 9, 10, 98, 102,
  108–10, 132
electric shock 38
emergency doctor services
  14, 170
emotional upset
  and abdominal pain 50
  and bladder control 62
  and breath holding 72–3
  and encopresis 89–90
encopresis 89–90
enuresis (bedwetting) 62–3
epilepsy 91
  and choking babies 34
erythema infectiosum 80
eye drops
  administering 19–20
  for hay fever 118
eye infections, conjunctivitis
  19–20, 88
eye injuries 15, 39
eyesight problems 110
  squint 153

face, bumps on the 31
facial swelling 54
febrile convulsions 92–3
feet
  athlete's foot 61, 132, 147
  flat feet 111
  itchy 132
'Fever Strip' 3
fevers 2–7, 79–82
  chickenpox 2, 11, 12, 80
  febrile convulsions 92–3
  and fluid intake 6, 167
  incubation period 2, 79
  keeping the child cool 7,
    21
  and kidney infections 136,
    137
  measles 80, 129–30
  mumps 81
  nursing during the night
    6–7
  paracetamol treatment 4,
    5–6, 57, 79, 93
  and rashes 10, 12
  scarlet fever 81
  and sore throats 151
  sponging treatment 4–5,
    79, 93
  symptoms 2, 80–1
  taking your child's
    temperature 3–4

and viral illnesses 167
  vomiting and dehydration
    167–8
  whooping cough 81
fifth disease 80
fingers, fractures 40
first aid kits 25–7
fits 91–3
flat feet 111
flu (influenza) 56, 131
folic acid 153
food
  allergies 53–4
  eating problems 105–8
  gluten-free 83, 84
food poisoning 113
foreskin problems 112
fractures 39–40, 47, 138
fungal infections
  athlete's foot 61, 132, 147
  ringworm 147–8
  thrush 133, 145, 157–8
  Tinea versicolor 148

galactosaemia 141
gastro-enteritis 49, 100,
  113–15, 167
German measles see rubella
glue ear 53, 98, 103
gluten enteropathy (coeliac
  disease) 83–4
GPs (general practitioners)
  170–1
  consulting
    and allergies 55
    and coughs 94
    and febrile convulsions
      92–3
    and headaches 119
    and insect stings 29
    and migraine headaches
      142
  and diagnosis
    asthma 59
    childhood fevers 5–6, 12
    meningitis 140
    rashes 10–12
    viral illnesses 166
  and emergency care 14,
    170
  and home visits 170
  homoeopathic 86–7
  and immunisation 130
  and medical care on
    holiday 16, 171